A MANIFESTO

HEALING A VIOLENT WORLD

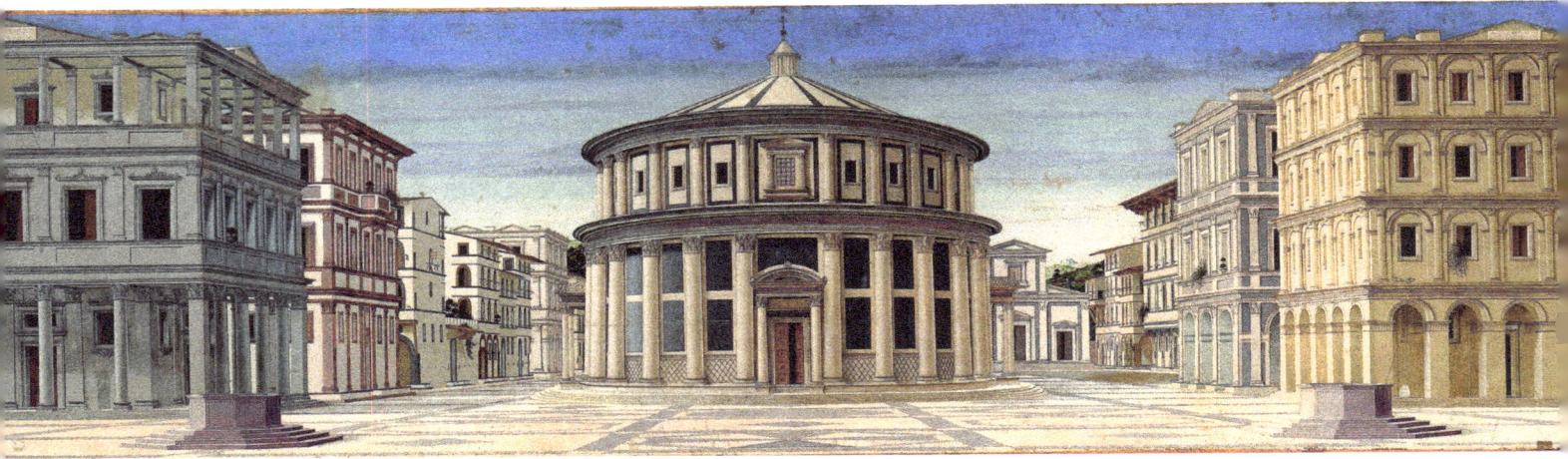

The Ideal City by Piero della Francesca, c.1415–92.

A MANIFESTO
HEALING A VIOLENT WORLD

Richard F. Mollica

Poems by **Marjorie Agosín**
(Translated from the Spanish by Celeste Kostopulos-Cooperman)

Essays by
Charles Figley, Nisha Sajnani, Christopher Mollica
and **Hanna Solomon**

Original artwork by **Nisha Sajnani**

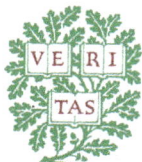

Harvard Program in Refugee Trauma

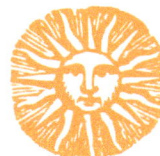

Solis Press

The Harvard Program in Refugee Trauma (HPRT) has pioneered the health and mental health of survivors of mass violence and torture, refugees, and traumatized communities worldwide over the past four decades.

Image credits: cover and page ii © Art Collection 3/Alamy Stock Photo; pages 1, 11, and 21 © Nisha Sajnani

ISBN: 978-1-910146-34-7

Published by Solis Press, PO Box 482, Tunbridge Wells TN2 9QT, Kent, England

Web: www.solispress.com | *Twitter*: @SolisPress

CONTENTS

DEDICATION

For all our mothers who gave us birth and nurtured ourselves and the world

Aster, Frida, Geni, Irene, Karen, Rakhee

PREFACE

Charles Figley

TRAUMAS ARE EVERYWHERE. OUR reactions to traumatic events and their memories are known and managed. We can now count the trauma because we know what to look for. The healing comes when facing the unhealed memories in the wake of trauma. Today, we know how stress affects the body, including the brain, and how best to mitigate that impact. Stress and the psychoneuroimmunological connections to illness require us to take stress seriously.

Trauma psychology and traumatology enable us to understand the risk and protective factors in managing traumatic stress reactions. But we do not know how to prevent and manage the causes of trauma. While traumatic stress impacts our mind in complicated and lasting ways; healing takes longer. How we heal a traumatized world is all about this book; what you are reading. I want to prepare you for reading this book.

We, the contributors to this volume, declare that **the world is hurting and needs to be healed and that structural and systematic change is needed to reduce violence**. The three manifestos, together with the sentiments of poetry, are produced to awaken your sense of healing. The urgency is obvious. This preface welcomes you to read this book mindful that the authors offer the manifestos under the shadows of crisis.

The manifesto for healing comes at a time in which the United States and places around the world are undergoing extraordinary political changes. These changes reflect and are reflected by the growth of economic inequity. The changes also come in the form of lower numbers with health-care coverage, compared to the past. Add to this, in 2018 alone, the high number of widespread, multiple, high-impact natural disasters and terrorizing shooting events. Collectively,

these events and conditions lower our sense of safety and confidence in the future.

Manifesto I recognizes the trauma around us. *Manifesto I* calls attention to our need to heal a violent world and what it takes to make that happen. Healing involves relief of suffering. The healer, then, like the first responders, runs towards the trauma, toward the people in need. Just as the sources of stress and methods of coping among all of us vary greatly, *Manifesto I* is about healing a cruel and violent world, one person at a time, through one healing practitioner at a time. The consequences of high doses of stress on people are well known, treatable, and preventable. Healers are the stars of *Manifesto I*. This is reflected in Marjorie Agosín's poem, "A Woman Dreams Between the Thresholds," an ode to the amalgam of all females who have survived trauma including and especially gender trauma; trauma imposed because of the gender of the harmed. The "invisible wounds" of gender-based violence manifesting in dread, sadness, and discouragement. This poem also wisely notes that all people helped by healers are also touched by the "grace of truth." She suggests that all human beings are able to create with the survivors, through deep listening to their trauma stories, a "maker of words, seeker of bodies, dreams of stories, weaver of justice."

In *Manifesto II*, Richard Mollica asserts hope to deal with the enormity of our current crisis. Through a new reality, the necessity of hope emerges. But the new reality requires the awareness of a violent, destructive, and heartless world for a new better world to emerge. It emerges as the healer and the healing person embrace the trauma – physical or mental – with courage to generate love and caring. The *Manifesto* recognizes the shared pain of the caregiver and the cared embedded within the historical context of the Wounded Healer. Healer and patient share their *woundedness*. But it acknowledges that out of this shared pain must come shared beauty to help transcend the pain. And with transcendence comes love, adaptation, appreciation, and sustainability. Healing from violence leads to familial and collective healing, and post-traumatic growth for the person, the family, and the community. The themes of *Manifesto II* are reflected in the poem by Marjorie Agosín. She offers expressions of appreciation for human services providers and caregivers of all types. Listening openhearted and wise, the healer unseals the sealed-up words and gives flight to unwanted emotions connected to words of pain. The healing practitioners listen, listen more, and listen again to all shades of trauma expressed in diverse forms, representing uncovered memories. This takes very hard work and commitment. Collectively, *Manifesto II* and its poetry provide the chorus of a song in honor of healers. The lyrics are about sacrifice and being in harmony with the pain of the healer that is the pain of the healed.

Manifesto III, the final manifesto by Richard Mollica, is a cry to embrace the healing power of justice. Healing builds on justice that gives hope to the healer and the healed. This manifesto declares that the foundation of justice is beauty. Beauty enables harmony and symmetry to lower stress and avoid future harm. This symmetry facilitates fairness that is in harmony with nature and stands in stark contrast to injustice. Injustice is "ugly." It lacks beauty and empathy. It is without harmony and symmetry. Injustice is inevitably associated with instability and insecurity at the personal and social levels. In contrast, justice leads to healing through love, respect, and safety. We know that "just" communities have the best chance of its citizens living together harmoniously in mutually beneficial ways.

The physician, Dr. Mollica, and the poet, Professor Agosín, in their wonderful assemblage of prose and poetry take us on a journey in this time of global crisis to *The Ideal City* of the Renaissance painter, Piero della Francesca. They reveal an often "hidden truth" and sometimes directed at perpetrators in our violent world: "The object of love's desire is beauty, beauty is justice, and justice leads to personal happiness and social harmony." The manifestos and poetry are a call to action for all of us to commit to creating a just and beautiful world free of violence. But healing the world requires first that we heal ourselves and work on remaining healed. Healing requires time. **Make time to heal.**

MANIFESTO I

HEALING A VIOLENT WORLD

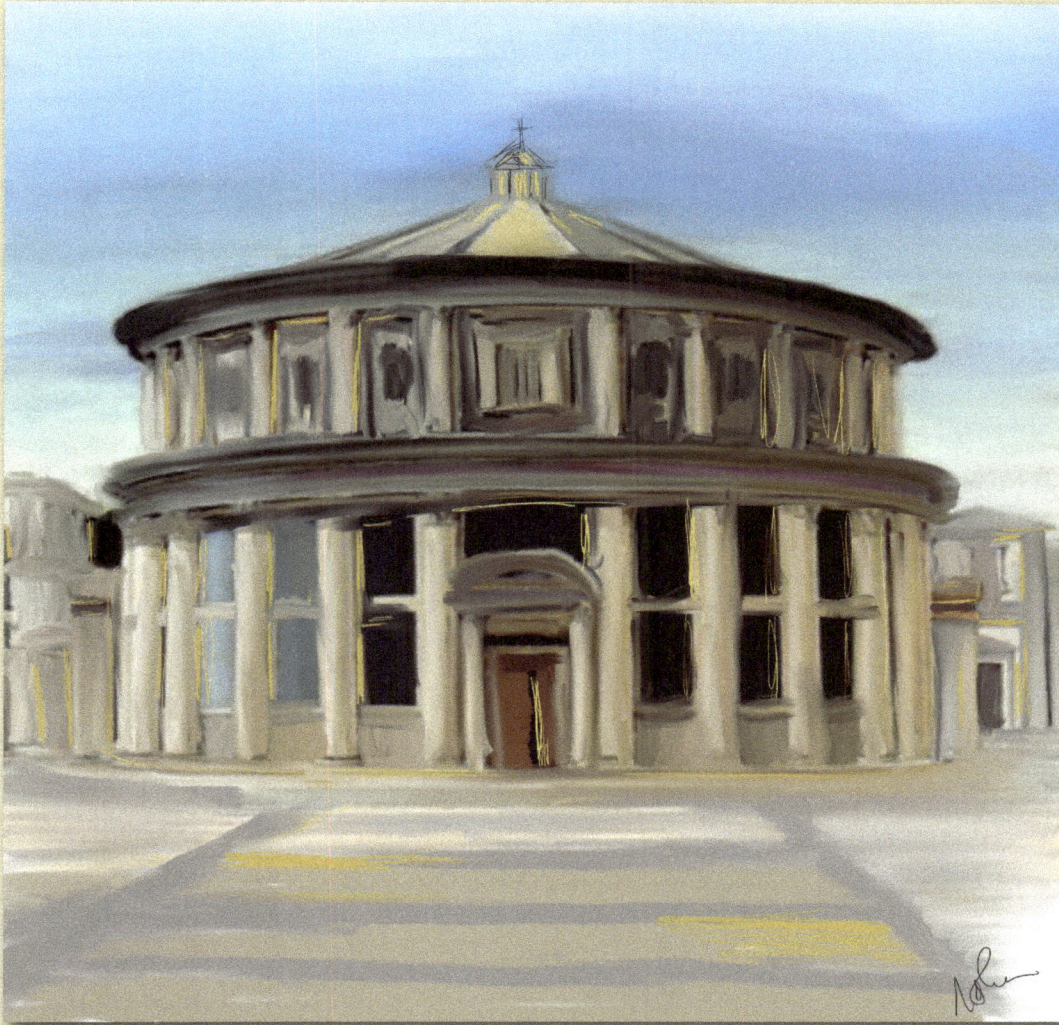

On our journey to the imperfect ideal city

MANIFESTO I

HEALING A VIOLENT WORLD

Richard F. Mollica

S EEING REALITY CLEARLY, WE observe that the world is awash in a sea of physical and mental suffering due to human cruelty. While at times this vision seems too much to bear, we do not give up on our dream for a more loving and peaceful humanity. Seeing reality clearly means that in this new age of global communication, the pain and suffering as well as the joys of each and every human can be heard by every other human being without censorship or the control by political and social forces that in the past and present rationalize and falsify the extent of man's cruelty to man. This new and original power of seeing gives us a technology of observing and changing the world comparable to that of the Italian Renaissance discovery of perspective by Filippo Brunelleschi, Leon Battista Alberti, and Piero della Francesca who moved us away from the flat two-dimensional images of the ancient and medieval world.

SEEING REALITY CLEARLY, we can no longer accept a world with more than forty nations in civil conflict and over one billion (i.e., one-sixth of our world citizens), harmed by mass violence. Torture is still widely accepted and is at epidemic proportions. Domestic violence, child abuse, and culturally sanctioned violence toward women, children, and persons of different gender and racial orientation are a plague on our planet. The trafficking and sexploitation of women and small children, including infants and pre-school-aged kids, are becoming thriving multi-billion-dollar industries. The commercial exploitation of youth and child labor and the economic oppression of the poor remains a financial pillar of many societies. The planet itself, which gave birth to all life forms, is selfishly destroyed.

UNAFRAID, we declare that uncontrolled human aggression and greed is a cancer on our world body that must be cured. As medical practitioners we affirm that modern medicine not only has the right, but the moral obligation to address human cruelty and violence as the leading cause of illness and death. The shocking silence in our medical schools, health, and public health institutions and among our healing community is so loud, it is deafening.

UNAFRAID, we affirm as healers of every type – community elders, religious, and spiritual healers, traditional healers and shamans, holistic medical practitioners, medical and mental health practitioners, counselors, teachers, artists, and all the human-oriented professions – that we can make a difference and reduce the pain of suffering from human cruelty.

1 THE GOAL OF HEALING has always primarily been the relief of human suffering. The healer must embrace with ardor this primary principle and subordinate the now dominant ambitions of speed and the obsession with the power of machines and molecules.

2 WE DECLARE THAT the patient is a beautiful living organism who freely acts and loves in a family and a community and is not an isolated body part or a disembodied mind. The healer must have a relationship with the man, woman, or child and their social and cultural context. Otherwise, human cruelty will continue to freely operate as a pathogen.

3 THE HEALER WILL understand that humiliation is the major instrument of human violence which is systematically applied to others to annihilate the individual, their family, and society. We must relinquish the myth that most violence is a random action perpetrated on an unsuspecting victim. Humiliation creates hopelessness, despair, anger, and revenge (often existing together) in the violated person. Humiliation must be acknowledged, and its victim released from its tight grip.

4 SCIENCE HAS REVEALED that at the moment violence strikes, the biological, psychological, social, and spiritual power of self-healing is activated. Today, many healers and social agents set up barriers that dampen the self-healing response. The pathway to recovery is filled with the roadblocks of human design and creation. Modern-day healers will do better to imitate their ancient Greek and Roman counterparts who followed the medical practice called *Vis Medicatrix Naturae*, that is, "the path of natural healing." These early physicians intimately knew the life course of an illness and gave hope to the patient through their knowledge and support of the self-healing process.

5 ALL HUMAN BEINGS embody the biological miracle of empathy, a wondrous power that enables us to identify oneself mentally with all other persons or objects of our contemplation. Sadly, empathic failure in human actions, including public policies and practices, is a core feature of violence and aggression. *Empathophilia*, the core of our empathic selves, needs to emerge as a centerpiece of our behaviors in our homes, schools, medical and professional institutions, public places, and public policies.

6 WE GLORIFY THE SURVIVOR of violence because of their heroic struggle to survive human violence, cruelty, and degradation. We strongly combat anyone who barbarically blames the victims or considers them guilty of criminal acts and subjects them to shame, social ostracism, and even death – especially those men and women who have been sexually violated.

7 WE GLORIFY THE HEALERS who, at great sacrifice to themselves materially and emotionally, engage in the case of traumatized persons worldwide. Through their compassionate and courageous work, they willingly suffer the pain of their patients as they engage in their therapeutic efforts. These healers in some situations risk their lives to help others, and in all cases accept upon themselves the victims' pain as their pain. In many communities of the world, these are the unheralded giants of the medical community. They need and appreciate our support and we joyfully give it to them.

8 THE TRAUMA STORIES of the survivor and their healers need to be collected and archived for all to read without censorship. Since the beginning of our humanity, these stories present an evolving history of survival and healing, teaching all of us how to cope with the tragic events of everyday life. The failure to collect and archive these stories denies us the opportunity to prevent a future generation of violence.

9 ONLY THROUGH IMAGINATION can healing occur. Healing is the imagination to heal. The survivor and the therapist create within themselves the image of a whole and complete human being who has shed the pain and suffering of the illness state caused by human cruelty. We will sing of wellness, resiliency, and a life full of love and friendship. We will sing of a world no longer tainted by human degradation and violent aggression.

10 EXCEPT IN BEAUTY there is no healing. Beauty is the salve and ointment that creates our healing space and healing relationships. Beauty is the preeminent healing medium that allows all physical, sociocultural, and spiritual forces to flow like the River Nile bringing all of the life-giving elements to the people of ancient Egypt. But many humans want to destroy beauty because of envy and a jealousy of its purity and innocence. Modern medicine wants to have with beauty a master–slave relationship. Realizing this, we will fight against all institutions and practices that are vulgar, ugly, sterile, and demoralizing. On this point, science reveals that beauty is healing's greatest ally.

11 AT THE START of this new century we are clear that the empathic circles formed by human beings need to be greatly expanded to include more of us. Everywhere we turn we find that the family, which is supposed to be a zone of love and affection, is filled with violence and child abuse. How can we consider all others as our brethren if we routinely harm our own family members? Worst of all, in most places, societies condone this behavior as normal. Family violence is not normal and is not acceptable. This failure at non-violent intimate relationships does not bode well for us holding back our aggression towards strangers outside our kinship groups. The fight against cruel degrading human behavior must begin with positive changes in the home!

12 WE WILL CALL a social myth the popular belief that acts of social justice and social healing from violence can occur without concern for personal healing. The desire for justice is embedded within the hearts and minds of all victims of violence and this reality must be openly acknowledged and supported by society.

On our journey to the new Ideal City, we will find at its end not the perfect environment of Piero della Francesca devoid of people, but one filled with human life. All of us can now see the dirty little secrets and ambitions of violent perpetrators who are actually few in number but use their money and power to harm the majority. We affirm that the world's magnificence can be fully realized, sustained, and protected from our human impulse to hurt and destroy all that is beautiful.

A WOMAN DREAMS BETWEEN THE THRESHOLDS

Marjorie Agosín

You could have been her
The girl amid the rubble
The girl dissolved by the haze of fire and hatred
But, you were not her.

You turned the corner of good fortune
Luck and its premonitions accompanied you.
But, could you have been her?
The girl amid the rubble?

Anne Frank sleepwalks through the streets of Amsterdam
Dressed in blood and gold.

You could have been the girl from Pakistan
With a bullet wound in the head
Punished for wanting to read, to write and to be.
You could have been that woman
On the corner steeped in wrath.
Time and again her husband beat her in the night
Joined together for so many years
By the persistence of his assaults.

It wasn't your turn, said the neighbor
Who thought about denouncing you at midday
When the Santiago city police
Came looking for you.

But you were not there
You had gone to speak with the surf
Were recently learning how to
Revive the soul
You always approached the sea as the universe
You and the sea
The sea and you
Linked in a symphony of generous words
Because you believed in wonder and in the magic of kindness.

And on the road you encountered an old toothless woman
Who told you heroic and fragile stories.
Did you listen to her words?
Or was it your love that saved you?
You listened to her with the wisdom of an older child
And you and she traveled along a map drawn in Sorrow
She told you that her village no longer existed
That only the geography of pain marked her face
And you kissed her fallen eyelids
Her hand like a burned and wounded forest.

And perhaps you never arrived at the city of Sarajevo
But imagined it on a canvas of anger
Or in a poem dressed in pain.
Perhaps someone told you that before searching for food
The women painted their lips in red and purple
And clothed the children with pages from books
Dostoyevsky, Victor Hugo, Neruda
Everyone clothing the children in memory and war
To dispel the horror on the face
To aim for beauty and not oblivion.

And when you heard the word, Srebrenica
Your body bristled with terror.
What could be done with the magnitude of hatred?
What could be done with the invisible abundance of love?

They had told you so many things
And you were not in the cities of fear.

Your story was simply another.

Bosnia was just an illusion
You had heard about Cambodia
And Vietnam
About Rwanda where the women embroidered
The names of their dead on their dresses
And Argentina where the women embroidered
The names of their missing children in their scarves.

Did someone tell you about the disappeared?
They were your age
They enjoyed going to cafés and singing at midnight
About the things of love
They played guitar
They sang the International
They did not fear the police
They just loved poetry.

But you did not go to the café
That night you covered other distances
You settled for the still frailty
Of an open book, like a serene leaf
From a festive magenta autumn.

When they called at the door you were not there
Your terrified mother with the unkempt hair
Came out and denied your whereabouts.
But you could have been there
You could have been the housewife of Belgrade
The cellist from Sarajevo
The disappeared girl in Buenos Aires
The child soldiers of Cambodia
The old woman raped in Bosnia
The one who wove blankets for her dead
The one who lost her voice and history
Until you came to sing it.

And what was history?
A game of chance?
A game of one type of cruelty over another?
Or perhaps the possibility of empathy?
Of finding beauty amid the hopelessness
The honor to call them by their names
The forgotten ones
The disappeared
The mutilated
The ones erased by history.

You refused the silence of the unjust
You opened their lips and their words
You learned to speak with the dead
To listen to their footsteps
And to save them a place at night
You were a Bridge and a Gaze
You were an open heart
Never sealed by cruelty.

One day you left with your voice hanging on your shoulder
Like a poet carrying bread
And you found yourself
Without crossing thresholds or borders
You were the little girl from Bosnia
That they raped and later scattered among the rubble
And she also cried out because you recognized her
Or perhaps you were one of the widows from northern Chile
Who searched for some little bones
A hand, a shoe, a flower between the words of the dead.

And each time you came back more clearly
They confused you with the angel of justice
The angel of memory
The angel of empathy.

But you looked around
And gathered histories
You embroidered them with the lighter side of your heart
And you did not look at the void
Only at the zones of pain.

A light was also there
Memory also persisted, there in the darkness
And you saw a resemblance in everyone
To the child soldier
To the young girl in Bosnia
And to the seeking mother.

And you found yourself in them
And they lived again in you.

In the night
You listen to them
And fill the celestial dome with stars from all the heavens
It seems that you have named them
It seems that the angels of hope
Mapped trails for your eyes.

You have received the grace of truth
You are all of them
And they are you.

Maker of words
Seeker of bodies.

Dreamer of stories
Weaver of justice.

(Translated by Celeste Kostopulos-Cooperman.)

MANIFESTO II

HEALING THE HEALER

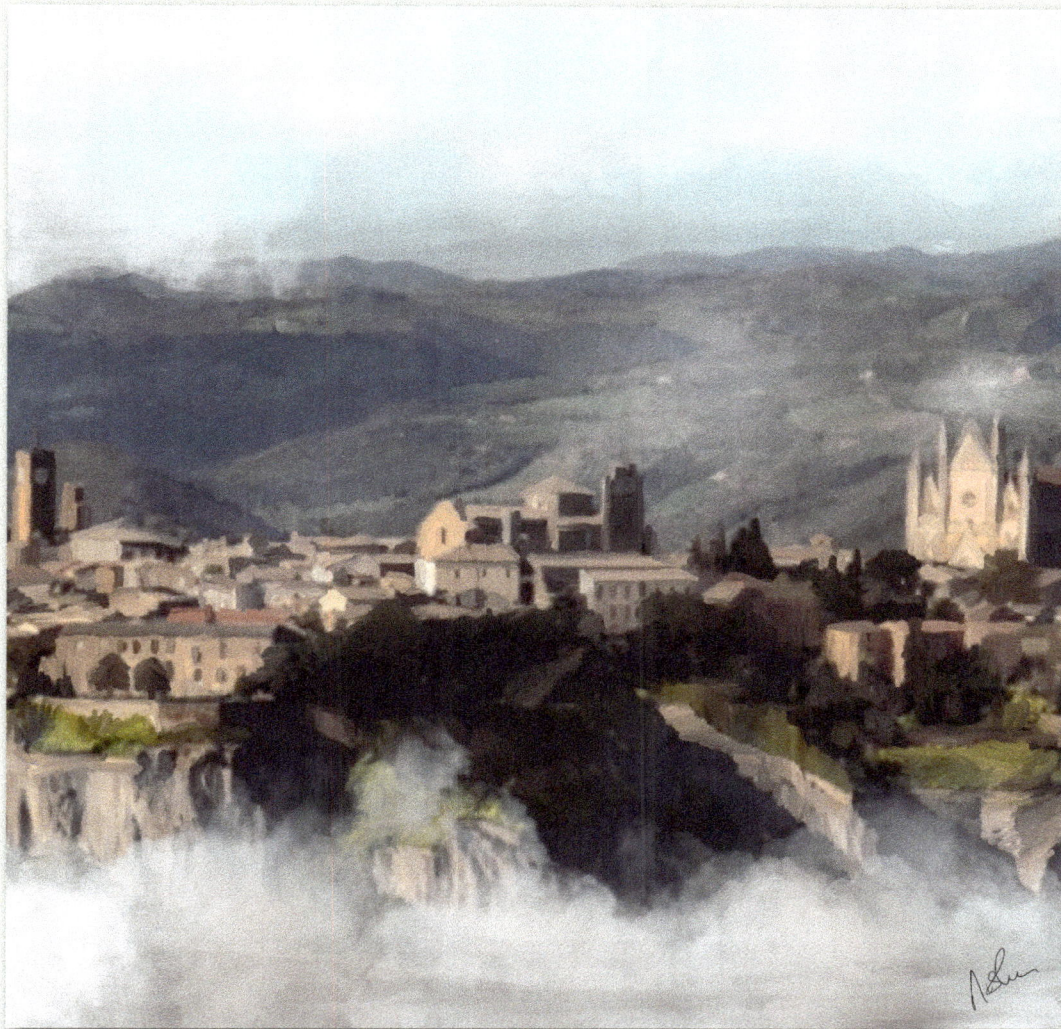

There was so much light in that city beloved by all

MANIFESTO II

HEALING THE HEALER

Richard F. Mollica

W E SING OF OUR healers and their clients who are the treasure of our world. Without health and well-being, people
have no freedom to escape from the tragedies and struggles of everyday life in order to create a new and better world. We are
in need of our treasure. We sing of those who have the courage to live
with tumors, wounds, broken limbs, broken minds, and other major
and unspeakable horrors that inflict on us pain, suffering, and ultimately death. Since the snake whispered into Melampus the secrets of
the world's natural medicines, the healer has united with the sick and
the afflicted to create a dream and realize a fantasy that two persons
in a shared empathic partnership within their life and their community can create a new reality.

We sing sadly that the sick person's pain is the healer's pain and
that nobody can truly know the reality of another. We sing proudly
that mankind since time immemorial has created sacred spaces and
environments to allow this wide gap to be closed. And that the god
Aesculapius has given the healer sanctity to touch all parts of the
body of man, woman, and child as well as entry into the conscious
and unconscious mind and soul of the sufferer. The sick know that
the healer is completely devoted to their welfare and that the healer
has forsaken money, power, and status as their primary preoccupation
and reward.

Healers go to the grave, poor men and women because of their devo-
tion and love for the patient, and love of medicine. But ultimately, we
sing joyously and loudly in chorus together that all healing has beauty
as the object of its desire. For without beauty there is no healing. And
beauty is the aesthetic that defines the healer–doctor and client relationship, the healing habitat, the disease and the patient's well-being.
Truly, the healer and client in each encounter celebrates the vitality
and living energy of all things including our animal friends, the plants
that nourish us and the earth itself.

UNAFRAID, we acknowledge that the healer is a *wounded healer*
achieving their cures in great agony and with stress on their bodies

and with a soul aching from the penetrating knife of disease. Sepsis, suppurating wounds, cachexia, tumors, parasites, HIV/AIDS, viruses, depression, hypomania, broken bones, and a million other ailments attacking living organisms from the inside and the outside. Great healers know each and every one of the illnesses well and, like old friends, follow them closely along their natural course to recovery or death. The ancient Romans called this *Vis Medicatrix Naturae* – the natural way. And like an old friend, disease asks the healer to pay a price in order to pursue the healing relationship no matter the outcome.

UNAFRAID, we acknowledge that the healer is a ***wounded healer*** achieving his and her cures bewildered and overwhelmed by a violent world. Something is wrong with the world; this cannot be denied. A never-ending stream of genocide, beheadings, mass murders, famine, poverty, racism, sexism, slavery, domestic violence, and trafficking wash across our human experience in an exponential way.

The healer waits at the riverbanks of a flood caring for a child and in a refugee camp listening to tens of thousands bearing unspeakable stories of human aggression. Healers cannot bear too much reality as they enter into a makeshift surgical suite in a devastated town in Syria or the Congo or a devastated hospital in a shantytown named after a number.

UNASHAMED, we declare that out of the healer's woundedness it is revealed that *"the body is our paradise, and the mind and soul the flowers and the garden of our humanity."* It is now our time to protect the sacred covenant that binds the healer and the healed together.

1 ALL LIVING THINGS are composed of the same genetic material tied in a grand unity, cell by cell. Ancient bacteria form the basis of our very mitochondria that energizes all life. Let no-one create a hierarchy of life forms so that one living organism can dominate another, or a healer dominate a patient, or the patient dominate a healer.

2 NO CHILD IS BORN AN EMPTY SLATE devoid of the social experiences of their ancestry. Hundreds of thousands of mirror neurons in the brain link us to our historical past. No longer can we laugh at Professor Carl Jung as a Lamarckian theorist, believing he had falsely proven that a collective unconsciousness binds all living things into a single unity. Now we can scientifically affirm that the child is born with the knowledge and strength of generations of survival as well as the fears and weaknesses of generations of violence and abuse directly transmitted to the infant. The healer and patient must always remember Michel Foucault, the great

French philosopher as he remarked, *"the body is imprinted by history."*

3 EMPATHY IS A BIOLOGICAL MIRACLE uniting all living creatures and the planet earth itself. Every human being can find love, affection, and caring in every other human being no matter the age, race, ethnicity, culture, gender orientation, or geographical location. Empathy is the foundation of all healing, but it comes at a cost. Little by little, healers accumulate within themselves the pain and suffering of their patients, building up a heavy weight of distress the healer can no longer bear. If we believe that empathy heals, then we must believe in *self-empathy* called *self-care*.

4 WE PRAISE THOSE healers brave enough to enter into the family life of those with serious emotional problems and disabilities. The broken mind is frightening to all, even the healer, since it is impossible for anyone to fully appreciate and understand the suffering caused by delusions, psychosis, hypomania, and severe depression. The burden of potential and real suicide on the healer is unimaginable. Healers are especially vulnerable when they have to confront traumatic life experiences in the patient's life including childhood sexual abuse, rape, gender-based violence, and domestic violence. Those brave healers who care for refugees and other survivors of extreme violence, such as torture, are to be commended. Nothing is more painful to a human being than to witness another human being hurting others. And we now know the pain that comes with the harm inflicted on animals, plants, and the earth itself. All call out for help, but few listen.

5 HOPE CAN BE A VERY WEAK HEALING CONCEPT that needs to be redefined. It is often used to "hedge one's bet" that the patient will get better. The concept of hope today hides and obscures the true meaning of prognosis in which the healer has lived with the illness over time and has a good handle on the medical outcome. Hope can only have value if the healer and patient are committed to work together over time as long as it takes to achieve a cure. *"I hope" must be transformed into "I will ... ."* An army general heading into battle never says to the troops, *"I hope we can get safely to the other side of the river."* The healer must always say (if true) that, *"we will succeed in conquering this illness."*

This comment requires consistent commitment, knowledge, and skills with a deep knowledge of the natural course of the disease. *I will* has transformed *I hope* into a new and powerful healing force.

6 WE CONDEMN THOSE healers who participate in acts of abuse of their patients, the patients' families, and their communities. The hypocrisy of proposing to patients diagnoses and treatments that harm needs to be exposed. Nothing can replace the **Golden Rule,** where *the healer treats the other as he or she would want to be treated.* We condemn the tacit acceptance of health disparities, racial biases in medicine, use of pointless procedures, and surgeries to gain financial benefits, shock treatment except in emergencies, restraining the mentally ill in straitjackets and chains, and the overdosing of patients with mind-numbing, diabetes-generating psychiatric drugs.

7 LET US ACCEPT FULLY and enter into the debate: "*Are laboratory tests, procedures, and surgeries an extension of the healer's senses, or are they a replacement of their senses?*" The healer has at their disposal all of the senses, even taste. Not too long ago the doctor tasted urine to check for diabetes or smelled the discharge of a wound. Some say a robot or a computer can replace the doctor. Certainly, those machines can avoid the emotional impact of an empathic partnership. But certainly, the senses enrich and deepen the therapeutic power of *the doctor–patient relationship.*

8 LISTENING, UNDERSTANDING, AND DEEP APPRECIATION (LUDA) is the foundation of the doctor–patient relationship. A universal truth exists – all patients love to be listened to about their problems. Deep listening is an *art* that needs to be practiced. LUDA leads not only to rich insight into the possible diagnosis, but it also contextualizes the patient. The healers come to know the patient's culture, social life, strengths, and barriers to treatment. The large number of patients with a history of current and past traumatic events need LUDA in order to share their **trauma story**. The *trauma story*, often neglected and/or ignored, is at the center of all medical and psychiatric care. LUDA leads to *trust* and trust leads to a strong therapeutic partnership. A strong therapeutic partnership allows the patient's suffering to be fully revealed.

9 THE PATIENT IS BECOMING MUTE AND THE HEALER DEAF. In our busy, noisy world, the doctor interrupts the patient after twelve seconds and spends less than fifteen minutes in consultation with the patient. We find it abhorrent when healers do not look away from their computer screens at the patient, clicking off check boxes on an electronic medical record (EMR) instead of describing the patient in their own words. Today, physicians call patients on a cellphone while driving in their car about serious laboratory tests and even yell at the patient for being late regardless of the reason. We decry the *industrialization of modern medicine* where the patient is transformed into a *consumer*, cancer becomes a *product line*, and the healer receives *love notes* from insurance companies instantly after submitting an incorrect bill on the EMR.

We revolt against the thousands of check boxes that now define our patients, their illnesses, and their treatments in the new EMR. Here, 50,000 doctors can look at a patient's records instantaneously and 180 million patients are integrated into one huge database in a trend that is growing quickly. Rapid unification of *our* personal data has many advantages including the speedy sharing of data among health-care providers. However, open access to personal patient data is threatening patient privacy. Secret and private discussions of sexual violence, for example, between the healer and client have no place being recorded in a massive depersonalized EMR.

The potential for data mining is grave, where at a moment's click of a computer button a government or business can find out everything they need to know about millions of patients. The isolated body parts of modern medicine have now been broken up into ever smaller digitized data units and recorded.

10 WE ARE REPULSED BY THE UGLINESS AND STERILITY of many healing environments. Let us acknowledge that healing spaces create therapeutic relationships, mobilize healing forces, and produce special outcomes, sometimes miracles. Who can prove that the Holy Ghost and/or other spiritual forces are not operating within our modern hospitals and clinics? The transformation of our healing spaces into impersonal and ugly places herald a full-scale attack on the healer and patient is becoming increasingly common. In

Western medicine, you can easily match the social status of the patient by the filth and stench present at the clinic. Psychiatric hospitals and clinics throughout the world are especially prone to this reality. They exhibit everything from submarine-like steel rooms with computers and desks to patients chained like animals in full public display. If you walk into a clinic and/or hospital anywhere in the world and it is very ugly and offensive to you – *walk out*. Or if this is all there is available – be hypervigilant to see that you and your loved ones are getting good care. We acknowledge and praise the beginnings of a medical revolution to create islands of beautiful healing gardens for cancer patients, children, and the chronically ill in emergency rooms, hospitals, and clinics. Look to the hospital and clinical space and assess its level of beauty and sensitivity to your culture. This will reveal for you the overall quality of care. No detail in healing is too small. This is what the Italians call *la bella figura – the beautiful way*.

THE INESCAPABLE TRUTH can no longer be denied – all healers everywhere are injured through their healing work and by the world in which we all live together. Within their shared healing spaces, healers have been able to bear this pain. African healers, Buddhist monks, Tibetan priests, Latin American shamans, and the religious and secular modern medical practitioners throughout the world have known the emotional and physical ointments to place on their wounds. But the industrialization of modern medicine is widening the gap between healing and self-care. We are entering an *apocalyptic age* where the brutality of man's inhumanity is creating terrible diseases and pain of unspeakable proportions. The ordinary healer, always courageous, must now become a *hero* and *heroine* in the fight against disease, materialism, commoditization of medicine and the direct attack by industrial forces on LUDA and their *sacred healing environments*.

The healer first must acknowledge their vulnerability and their own wounds. The basic practices of self-care must be practiced including diet, exercise, stress reduction, and time well-spent with family and friends. Meditation, reflection, and awareness can lead to a diminution of pain.

We fully acknowledge and bear witness to the reality that an *empathic horizon* needs to be set as a primary goal. Patients and fellow healers are bound together on this journey to the horizon in a shared community of empathic reciprocity and respect. The healer and the patient can only find themselves by finding out the meaning of the other. This empathic connectedness is based on a conversation: a powerful discourse between the patient, the healer, the illness, and the world.

CONVERSATION is at the foundation of our civilization and all of medical care. Healers desperately need to be in conversation with their colleagues, patients, family, and community. Out of the healer's woundedness, everyone can share in a united immunity and therapeutic presence. Courageously, small groups of healers and patients within their beautiful, shamanistic, and sacred enclaves multiplied a million times over throughout our universe are making a difference. How wonderful it is that out of our woundedness we can all help to change ourselves, modern medicine, and the world.

CARRIERS OF LIFE

Marjorie Agosín

I
Generous, openhearted,
they practice the wise,
deliberate silence of those who listen.

II
Between the thresholds of the wind,
beyond fleeting
memory,
they listen to
the sealed up words,
the motions of silence.

III
They listen to
the sounds of war
because they know how
to hear between the silent
stories behind the walls.

IV
Generous and openhearted,
they understand the words of the wounded
and offer fear a refuge
they are like a festival
they are travelers of light.

MANIFESTO III

HEALING POWER OF JUSTICE

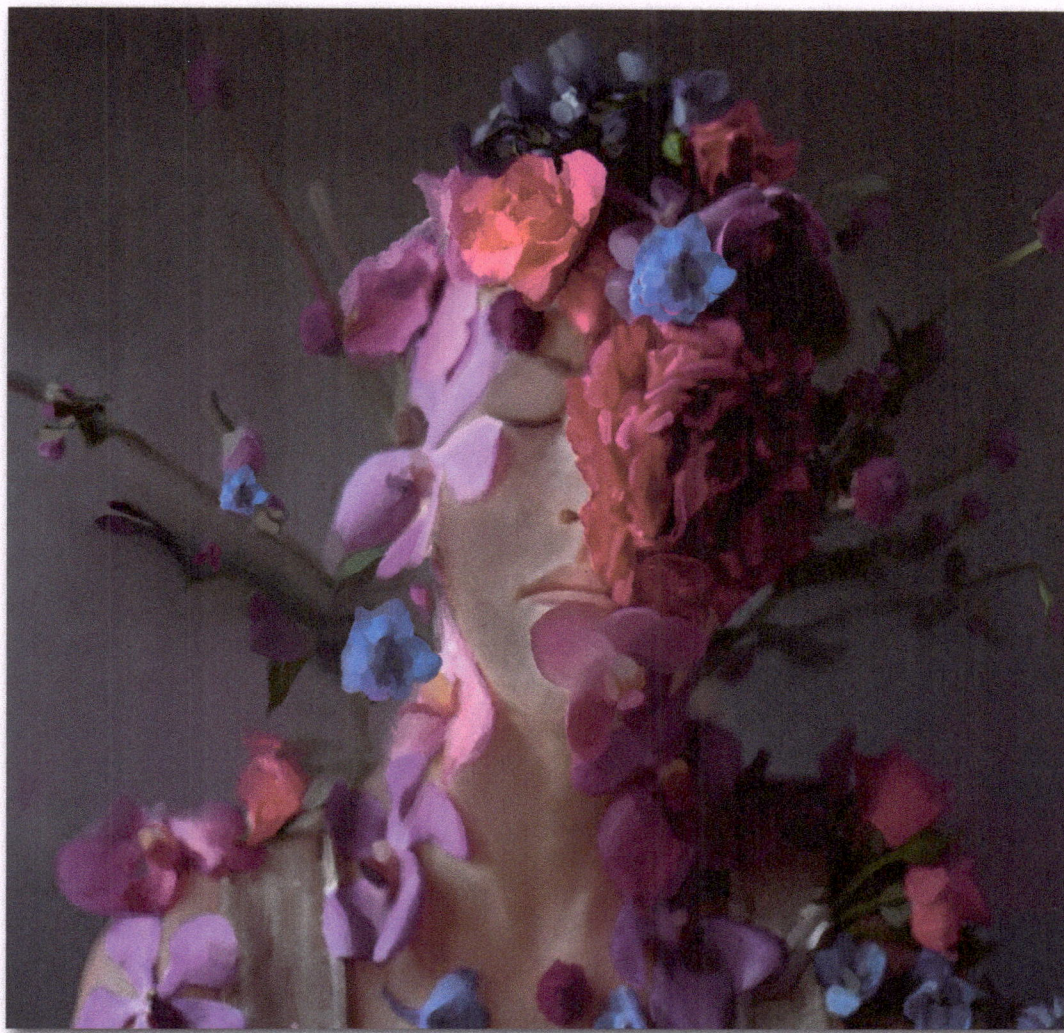

The body is our paradise, and the mind and soul the flower and garden of our humanity

MANIFESTO III

HEALING POWER OF JUSTICE

Richard F. Mollica

L ISTEN – WE LOUDLY DECLARE – THERE IS NO HEALING WITHOUT JUSTICE AND THERE IS NO JUSTICE WITHOUT HEALING. The world is awash in a sea of *violence* and *brutality*. Everywhere the world is bearing witness to unspeakable atrocities against human beings and nature. Genocide and ecocide are becoming all-familiar realities to the young who are facing despair and hopelessness. All civilized human beings throughout the world are paralyzed by the **enormity** of the challenge of changing the world to a more **peaceful** and **loving** environment.

IN SORROW we lament our long history of "*revolting injustice*" a term used by St. Augustine in the fifth century to describe the ongoing corruption and escalating decline of the late Roman Empire. Who cannot deny that we now live in an age dominated by "*might makes right*" and the "*big fish eating the little fish.*"

Gangs of criminals are running our governments and businesses. Painfully, we must acknowledge that our instruments of national and international laws are failing miserably to protect all living things from rampant destruction, exploitation, and the spread of poverty and diseases. Is it true what the early Greek sophists stated, "***Justice is in the eyes of the beholder,***" they said that "obeying laws renders us helpless to those who do not obey the law."

While many follow the prescribed laws in public, self-interest and greed dominate personal and corporate behavior. Just as health is intrinsically good – **injustice is a disease**. Injustice, because of its terrible negative impact on our personal and social lives must be avoided and fought against at all cost.

Our ancient ancestors in the West originally named justice with the Latin term: *justitia* – i.e., *righteousness* or *equity*. To the ancient, justice is at the heart of establishing an **order** and out of this order *beauty* and *harmony*. Its origins may have been derived from the ancient Egyptian goddess Maat. This goddess is seen holding a scepter in one hand and a symbol of an *ankh* (eternal life) in the other with an ostrich feather in her hair. Maat transforms into the Greek goddess Themis and her daughter Dike who in turn emerges as the goddess of justice, holding a sword in one hand and scales in the other. We embrace our origin myths and those of other cultures including India, China, and local indigenous people who gave justice a name, a face, and a standard of civilized behavior.

WE ACKNOWLEDGE that since the beginning of human history, the struggle for justice has been intense and often tragic. The Greek Titan Prometheus created mankind and gave human beings fire and they became civilized. A jealous Zeus condemned Prometheus to an eternal life of torment. He was tied to a rock and an eagle tore out his rejuvenating liver everyday for eternity. Prometheus must bear this horrible pain for being **kind and compassionate to human beings**. And when he was freed by Hercules, we see the frail and weak Prometheus in the great Etruscan bronze mirror of the sixth century BC leaning against Minerva (the Greek Athena), who is the symbol of justice and the nursing goddess of Roman mythology. Chiron, the centaur, made the ultimate sacrifice by offering to exchange places on the rock with Prometheus, suffering the same fate.

WE SING LOUDLY in praise of Chiron, the world's first physician and the teacher of Asclepius the Greek god of medicine. Chiron, through his compassion and selflessness as a medical doctor, offered himself as a sacrifice. Chiron is the model for all physicians who heal the world through the courage of sacrifice. Look up at the stars and you can see Chiron today looking down on us in the constellation Centaurus.

UNAFRAID, we declare that justice is a **beautiful thing**. Justice is *symmetrical*, it is *intricate*, it is a highly designed *aesthetic*, and a value system that creates a well-ordered, peaceful, and fair world. Justice through beauty creates health and well-being. Society and its people, its factories and farms, and the natural world flourish in a just world. In spite of all the competing theories of justice, it is clear that justice must be based upon *love* – for ourselves, for each other, and for our natural and physical world.

IN CELEBRATION of our desire to create goodness in our world, we declare that only out of *love* can we find and create beauty and justice in our everyday lives and in our violent and destructive world. It is our time to acknowledge, recognize, protect, and grow the sacred bond of love that binds justice and healing together into a **powerful force of human and social transformation**.

1 INJUSTICE MAKES US SICK. Treating human beings unfairly creates physical and emotional distress. It has been clearly established that the impact on health can be direct (e.g., criminality, pollution, enslavement, and domestic violence) or indirect (e.g., poverty), including all forms of economic oppression, and life-threatening and disabling actions. All injustices are a violation of human freedom, autonomy, and well-being no matter how minor a violation. Injustice is *brutish* and *ugly* because it causes a rupture in the peaceful order of things by tearing apart two basic rules: (1) People should not harm each other and (2) people should try to help others to the extent within their means.

2 WHEN HUMAN BEINGS "HURT" OTHER HUMAN BEINGS, the potential impact on health and wellness can be severe. All human beings experience *tragedy* in their lives. This is unavoidable. But when someone hurts another the health impact is terrible. Violent, traumatic actions of injustice such as rape, child abuse, and the atrocities of civil conflict and war lead to serious medical and mental health illness and even death. The violated person "*loses the world*". Everything they believe in about a *just* and *fair* world is destroyed. Humiliation is the main instrument of violent perpetrators that is used to cause the state of *humiliation*. Victims blame themselves; they are often socially stigmatized and even killed (e.g., in cases of rape). All survivors feel socially isolated.

3 WE PRAISE THE United Nations Declaration of Human Rights (probably the greatest document of justice written by mankind). It affirms the right to justice based on the universal principles of **equality, freedom of thought and expression**, and **access to the basic political and material needs** to lead a good and happy life. Unfortunately, in most societies **gross class inequalities, gender-based violence,** and **lack of political freedom** still exist. Political corruption, ethnic conflict, and civil war are rampant. Atrocities of a horrible nature are revealed daily without any punishment or containment. Beheadings, systematic rape of women and children, the massive global migration of refugees and migrants fleeing poverty and violence, and the genocide of indigenous people (e.g., Tibetans) seems to be on the rise.

4 WE CONDEMN THE ongoing neglect, destruction, abuse, and killing of our silent animal partners and all that exists within the world of *nature*. Many philosophers, such as the American transcendentalists, believed that a "*spiritual*" life exists in all of humans and that it can only be discovered through nature. Scientists have revealed the healing power of animals and the natural world in the care of the physically and mentally ill. We praise the fact that healing gardens are being built for patients who are terminally ill and in need of hospice care. Hospitals are being turned into beautiful healing environments; refugee camps are being transformed by the planting of trees, shrubs, and vines within every convertible space. All environments including terrible shantytowns, prisons, and refugee camps can be transformed into healing habitats.

5 WE ASSERT THAT all human beings have the right to **culturally effective health and mental health care** without the domination of the healing system by its political bosses. We condemn discrimination due to race, gender, sexual orientation, social class, and ethnicity. Neglect, disrespect, lack of access to medical care, excessive drug use, inferior and harmful treatments such as unnecessary surgeries, and seclusion and constraint of the mentally ill are wrongful practices that need correction.

The outdated World Health Organization's statement of health ("Health is a state of complete physical, mental and social well-being and not merely the absence of disease and infirmity") needs to be replaced by a **creative principle of personal autonomy**. There should be no excessive power, or privilege to the hospital or health and/or government insurance companies. We decry a patient being called a *commodity*, cancer *a product line* and the medical record a series of *check boxes*. Contemporary feminists in Gujarat, India, have come up with a new definition of health care: "Health is a personal and social state of balance and well-being in which people feel strong, active, wise, and worthwhile; where their diverse capacities and rhythms are valued, where they may decide and choose, express themselves, and move about freely."

No longer can we stand by when a patient is said to be healthy by physical examination and laboratory test, yet every day is beaten by their spouse or crushed under the daily weight of economic poverty.

6 *JUSTITIA* OUR BLINDFOLDED GODDESS who is holding the scales of justice is under attack. We state forcefully that justice is not equal to the law. Justice is *fairness*. Justice is a virtue related to "*goodness*" and "*beauty*."

In our modern world, justice may be manipulated with and controlled by the rich and powerful. Laws may be considered legal but not equitable or fair. In the human rights field dominated by lawyers, the healing of the violated victim is often neglected and/or completely ignored.

It has not been demonstrated, for example, that Truth Commissions, while carrying out a political purpose, also serve the personal healing of the oppressed citizens. In Bosnia, where testimony was offered in the courts by victims, the alleged perpetrators were released because they could not be convicted under the "*rule of the law.*" The Bosnian victims and their communities were devastated by these results. Many torture survivors are encouraged to give testimonies of gruesome stories in court only to be abandoned by the courts and their lawyers without treatment once the trial is over. While infectious diseases such as cholera or tuberculosis are not tolerated in United Nations refugee camps, neglect of the seriously mentally ill is common and rampant ongoing rape of refugee women, children, and young girls goes unchecked while we applaud the growing use of witness impact statements in court rooms, but much more needs to be done.

Justice can only be served if there is respect not only for basic human needs such as food, water, shelter, clothing, employment, education, and ongoing protection from physical harm, but also concrete attention to the physical, emotional, and spiritual well-being of the survivors. For way too long, the *emotional* (i.e., mental health) and *spiritual* needs of survivors have actively been pushed aside. Individuals and communities can languish in poverty and despair, and social mistrust, while lawyers argue their legal cases in the courtrooms.

7 WE WILLINGLY ENTER into the debate that there may be little, if no relationship between *social healing* and *personal healing*. Does the well-being of the community take precedence over the well-being of society's individual members?

When mass violence occurs, there is damage not only to individuals but to entire societies, indeed to the world. The victims of the September 11 attack and their families and friends suffered horrible losses, but even those of us who watched the television footage suffered, whether by experiencing depression, anxiety, a loss of faith in humanity, empathic overload, or emotional withdrawal. As a consequence, healing must occur not only within individuals but also within societies, with **society as the healing agent**.

Trauma sufferers need society's assistance in the self-healing process, and in turn they help society heal by sharing their stories, experiences, and wisdom. Personal and social healing are united in a reciprocal and mutually advantageous relationship. Through the journey of self-healing that each one takes, survivors can teach the rest of us how to recover from injury in a violent world.

8 THIS RADICAL SHIFT in society's view of the violated and traumatized persons must begin with the survivors themselves sharing their stories. The *telling* of their trauma stories is a key element in linking personal and social healing. The sharing of traumatic life events to truly interested listeners, especially those interested in *restoring justice* can pull storytellers out of their *isolation*, feelings of *shame*, and *humiliation*. For many, the telling of the trauma story is an integral element of personal healing. In a dialog and/or conversation, two people construct a mental canvass of events. Left to their own minds and thinking, the survivors can wander over their life history *undisciplined* and *unguided*. Storytelling to others has boundaries and limits. Together, the storyteller and listener are able to acknowledge the survivor's traumatic life events and together create a journey of healing and recovery. This new creative process can reorder the broken justice system. Paradoxically, it not only serves the survivor – but also the trauma survival and healing. This enhances resiliency and can help prevent future violence. A secret is now revealed, i.e., all stories are narrative of survival and healing – for the entire society.

9 A MAJOR FOUNDATION OF JUSTICE IS LOVE. In St. Augustine's concept of justice, *Divine Love* overrides all secular concepts of love. Human beings need to aspire to higher principles than the common desire to harm others out of self-interest, greed, fear, envy, revenge, and the political need for domination. In contrast, the ancient Greek philosophers who were agnostic about their Gods in their society described six forms of love:

- *Eros* – sexual love
- *Philia* – deep friendship
- *Ludus* – playful love
- *Agape* – a great love for everyone
- *Pragma* – long-standing love
- *Philautia* – self love.

Agape is the "love" greater than "love," i.e., the universal love that binds all human beings, the world of nature, and society together into a harmonious *beautiful* unity. *Justice is a virtue* according to Plato, the richest aspect of *goodness*. Through love of ourselves, our neighbors, and our larger universal life forces we can achieve a just world. The ultimate and simplest rule of justice is the "Golden Rule": you should treat others as you would like others to treat oneself. Many physicians believe the key to medicine is the "love of the patient." Certainly, the other side of the coin is "Do No Harm"! The Golden Rule and these basic medical attitudes are present in all societies and cultures.

10 AND THE MAJOR FOUNDATION OF JUSTICE is **beauty**. Justice is beautiful as it creates *harmony* and *symmetry* in the world that resonates with all animals, plants, and people. Injustice is *ugly* – it is a gaping injury and a wound on our social and natural world. Injustice cries out for restoration – sometimes injustice is a social and personal **cancer** that needs to be cut. At other times it needs a healing space or ointment. But this ugliness and disharmony demands treatment. Beauty is also associated with justice because it inspires creativity. Beauty pushes us into the realm of the transcendent and spiritual. It expands our love for ourselves and our fellow human beings and our natural environment. Beauty, expressed through works of art or found in the natural world, can strike deeply at all levels of our existence. On reflection, beauty can open us to the **truth**. A wise person can follow, for example, the wisdom of beauty and nature to behave politically in a *just* and *harmonious* way according to the *I Ching*. English poet John Keats (early 1800s) summarized it simply:

> Beauty is truth, truth beauty, – that is all
> Ye know on earth, and all ye need to know.

It is now revealed: THE OBJECT OF LOVE'S DESIRE IS BEAUTY, BEAUTY IS JUSTICE, AND JUSTICE LEADS TO PERSONAL HAPPINESS AND SOCIAL HARMONY.

It all comes together, **justice** and **healing**. One element cannot exist without the other. As we journey to *The Ideal City* of the great Renaissance painter Piero della Francesca, we acknowledge that human beings have a profound rejuvenating spirit capable of finding a deeper meaning in life. With great *beauty* in our lives, we create justice and happiness for all living creatures on our planet earth. The *power* of healing contributes to this great quest for justice. We seek out the Shining City on the Hill. In Piero's world, this *Ideal City is open to all who choose to enter.*

PSALM 85:10 COMPASSION AND TRUTH MET; PEACE AND JUSTICE KISSED

Marjorie Agosín

The ferocity of the winter had not
Yet arrived in the cities.

Like a sunflower, the fall with its colors
Still ruled the sky.

Couples played among the leaves.

While lovers dreamt
About luminous rivers
And love was like
The texture of water.

There was so much light in that city
Beloved by all.

Some children climbed among the trees
Wanting to collect stars.

But suddenly, upheaval gripped the streets.

Death arrived at the most unexpected places.
At a bar where people used to offer a toast
To the city of light.

At a concert hall where a piano
Shattered into a thousand pieces
Like abandoned bodies.

It was in Paris and in Istanbul

In New York City and
In a neighborhood in Kabul.

They were everywhere
And we were everyone.

The upheaval also erupted
In a marketplace in Beirut
Where women carried children
And sweet dried fruit,
And where pomegranates appeased faith.

The words fell silent.
Throats dried up.
Pianos split open in
A heartbreaking wail.
Language became vulnerable.

We didn't know how to name them.
The ones who were thirsty for death
Lost and without a compass.

The upheaval was not only there.
It was felt in the whole world
In houses big and small.

The sky cried ashes of tears.
The meadows were drenched in fall sunlight
And were blanketed by black clouds
That eclipsed the earth.

A young girl's head was cut off.
She could have been Dalila,
She could have been Marie
And her hair fell among the leaves
In the parks of Paris,
It fell in the markets of Beirut
Looking like a ring of fire.

They killed little Tatiana in mid-air.
Her doll also died in her hands
Both lost amid the rubble.
And the sky ceased being the sky.
The heavens became a shawl of tears
A howl, the scale of a sobbing universe.

And we wondered if this was our world
Or if perhaps it was another
If it was the other way around?

Or if we had entered the most evil zones
Where words are bereft of meaning.

And suddenly everything was immersed
In the deepest silence.
Only death
Among the streets
Among the boulevards
Among the cornices of Alexandria
And the narrow streets of Tunisia.

Death carried black banners
From so much bloodthirsty killing
It had also lost its breath and voice.
Death became entangled in itself
And fell in its own trap
The void
Of senseless pain
The carnival of deranged blood.

Death feared itself.
The earth also decided to swallow it.

And the children lay hidden
In the abandoned parks, perhaps dead
Among the leaves that turned
Ashen gray.

Look at the black cloud dancing in the world.
Look at the black cloud.

And where was Justice?
Had it gone away?
Had it moved to another place?

Where was the woman who carried
The tablet of hope?
Where was the noble goddess
Of bountiful generosity?
The woman who appeared in dark nights
To guide lost travelers?

And we ask ourselves if there will be
A lighthouse to give us shelter?
A place that will protect us?

A country?
A city?
A forest?

The world suddenly fell silent.
The universe stopped singing.

The crickets, the wind, the waves
Stopped bursting,
Stopped being.

Did we have to begin to name it again?
How would we be different from the past?

Suddenly Justice returned.
She appeared radiant and barefoot.
She had fallen asleep like all of us.
Ingenuous and sometimes comfortable,
Innocent and other times arrogant
In her innocence.
She also feared not being able to be as before.

Justice spoke and said:

There will be no vengeance or hatred,
Nor will there be oblivion.

We will return to play in the
No longer abandoned parks.

We will dance again in the hills
Of our cities.

We will go joyfully to the markets and
Our baskets will fill with the
Offerings that the earth grows and provides.
Barbarism will be transformed into beauty.
Justice will dress in strands as golden as the sun
Like the light that rules over the planet.

Children will not kill other children.
The children will play on seesaws, on swings,
And with the stars.

And Justice will be made with words
That will be words again.
Tolerance and solidarity
Empathy and goodness.

Affectionate words
Beautiful words
Fluorescent stars
Fireflies.

Justice disappeared within the foliage.

And suddenly the children appeared
Jumping on the leaves.
And a young girl said that
She liked to count the stars.

Another invited us to her home by the sea
Because the lighthouses had returned,
And the wise old women told
Stories on the rocks.

It seemed like the world had turned around,
It had returned to its place.

We decided to remain on the side of beauty.
To confide in the night and the day.
We decided to touch the light,
And attend the concerts of the
Water and the earth.

And imagine cellos like deep forests
And pianos like a cascade of living water.

We chose life
And the paths of the possible.

To embrace living symbols
To love the silver butterflies and the monarchs
To love the thunder and the storm
The abundance of stars and poetry.

Not to be afraid to live among those
Different from ourselves.

Justice suddenly appeared again
Without the weights
She had carried before.
She seemed like a floating bride,
Like a fairy predicting good signs.

Justice smiled,
Saying that this will be the road.

We will achieve more
When there is no more hatred or fear.
When oblivion makes way
For luminous memory.

And above all, when we will mend
The fallen bodies
The mutilated voices.
And the children's gaze
Like a river of fear.

We will achieve for the now
When the wolf talks with the lamb
Just as the ancients had written.
And when the light within you
Will be your safe harbor.

Before departing, Justice in all her
Beauty and lightness of being said:

There will be no more hostile roads of fear.
The cities will open
Their enormous, glorious avenues
With pedestrians walking confidently
Among the museums and cafés,
Among the concert halls and their homes.

And the sky will once again be
A galaxy of possible magnitudes.
The children will count the stars again
And draw the Milky Way.

Justice promised that beauty
Would bathe the fields with poppies
Where grenades and blood had once been.
And that the rain would cleanse
The universe.

Justice departed without weights.
She danced barefoot throughout the earth
And rose toward the sky.

(Translated by Celeste Kostopulos-Cooperman.)

MOMENTS OF REVELATION

Richard F. Mollica

THIRTY YEARS OF CARING for people exposed to extreme violence and torture have led to outbursts of scientific clarity. Italian philosophers call these *i momenti*, moments of revelation. These insights created this manifesto: *Healing a Violent World*. With modesty, as a medical doctor, I take on the challenging topic of ending human violence. Hearing thousands of trauma stories demands this effort. I would be acting in bad faith if I ignored this monumental task while my patients coped with atrocities of unspeakable horror.

The dictum my Italian immigrant father voiced, also a victim of violence, remains loud and clear, "Son, take on a problem you cannot solve." Now is the time. We live on the edge of apocalyptic annihilation through our destruction of the planet, its millions of living species and humankind itself through arsenals of nuclear, biological, and chemical weapons. The destructive nature of human violence is all around us extending from nuclear bomb-making in North Korea, cannibalism by rebel forces in the Democratic Republic of the Congo to epidemics of domestic violence in many countries and societies.

After the Twin Towers attacks in New York City on 9/11, I became aware of the aggressive and degrading conversations and practices that occur daily in our workplace, churches, and hospitals. While responding to the unfolding tragedy in New York after the terrorist attacks, to attend to the families of the victims of 9/11 and their medical caregivers, I was asked daily by both friends and strangers, "What can I do personally to help out with this tragedy?" And I spontaneously exclaimed, "Try to reduce the aggression in your everyday life towards everyone around you." The suffering impacting on me during my work in New York was so intense that it resulted in generating a new human skin very sensitive to all forms of human aggression. The pain of the victim of 9/11 became my pain; the pain of the many torture survivors I have treated has passed into my body and mind and become part of my life. This personal transformation led to a shocking realization that something was missing from far too many human interactions. This missing ingredient was empathy, the basic capacity to experience the physical sensation, emotions, and thoughts of another human being. The most disturbing experiences of my career now made sense as instances of empathic failure. The fact that people who are basically decent engage in harmful human practices and policies had blinded me to this truth. Normal people have a "will to deny" the physical and emotional suffering of others, thereby obscuring the true impact of their behavior.

Past voices of empathic failure that I cannot silence are loud and lingering in my mind. In the early 1990s, over 500,000 Cambodian refugees living in squalid prison-like conditions on the Thai–Cambodian border were finally going home. Our team spent many years trying to relieve their emotional suffering from losses of a genocide and the harsh decade-long deprivations, exposure to rape and physical violence in the refugee camps. In the midst of these camps of "hopelessness" and "despair," a mental health program was established by our team with the refugees themselves as healers. Hundreds had been trained as mental health workers capable of assisting in the repatriation process. But the United Nations (UN) Chief of Repatriation said no to the utilization of these well-trained Khmer health and mental health practitioners. Then in a moment of incomprehensible truthfulness he stated, "These people are just rocks. I'm going to load up these half million rocks and carry them in big trucks and dump them across the border." His response and officially sanctioned policy devastated our collective sense of shared purpose with our Khmer colleagues. With one single word, "no," this UN official ignored the traumatic history of the Khmer people. The rocks were returned impoverished to a devastated countryside.

At the time of the mass exodus from Vietnam, Laos, and Cambodia, at the end of the Vietnam War, I received a photograph from the Thai–Cambodian refugee camps of a Cambodian woman who had been captured by militia as she and her family fled into Thailand to escape the violence of the Vietnamese occupation of Cambodia. She was raped, both hands amputated, her husband tortured and killed along with two of her four children. She arrived desperate in the refugee camp. Our Khmer colleagues sent us her photo with a note on the back asking for clinical help since the "woman had lost her mind with grief." Finally, we had hard, clear documentation of the mental health needs of Cambodian victims of violence in the Thai refugee camps. This picture was brought to the Human Rights Director of a major private foundation and a request was made for mental health assistance for this woman, her family, and other Khmer survivors of torture and mass violence. After studying the picture, the response from the Director was a clear "no" because she stated that this woman had not suffered a human rights violation. Anger filled my mind, was I insane? How could a Cambodian woman who had experience such savagery not be a victim of a human rights violation? But according to the strict reading of existing international legal covenants at the time, sexual violence and rape were criminal acts and not crimes against humanity. Her other traumas were also considered criminal acts because they had been committed by a militia group. One wonders if this degree of empathic failure took a considerable degree of emotional energy; or maybe none at all. In any case, it resulted in the denial of a human tragedy.

There is nothing new about violence towards women and children. Domestic violence is rampant. It is a common condition everywhere no matter the relative wealth of a local community or a country. The "spoils of war," a term used to describe the rape and murder of women, young girls, and boys, goes back to the beginnings of recorded history. In 1988, our Harvard team along with Amnesty International published the first scientific study to reveal that sexual violence was used as the major torture of women globally. Until the extraordinary and courageous "speaking out" of Bosnian women during the late 1990s, sexual violence during violent conflicts was considered a "war crime," i.e., "business as usual during wartime." Through the efforts of Bosnian, and later Rwandan women, sexual violence was elevated legally to a "crime against humanity." In spite of these new laws, sexual violence continues unabated in places such as Sudan, Democratic Republic of Congo, and Syria. The children of rape and their mothers are neglected and receive little support and attention.

In refugee camps throughout the world, sexual harassment and outright rape is a common daily occurrence. This abuse occurs in spite of international safety and protection, food, water and shelter, and the prevention of infectious diseases. This gender-related violence was initially discovered by myself in the early 1990s when our Harvard team was conducting the first ever mental health study of a refugee camp. An enlightening and shocking experience occurred in the largest Cambodian displaced persons camp called Site 2 on the Thai–Cambodian border. Our team found each morning when we visited Site 2's makeshift hospitals, that the female nurses and patients were underneath their hospital beds. They told us they were hiding in terror from being raped each night from the soldiers hired by the Thai government to protect them. In dark, unlighted refugee camps today, women and children continue to live in fear of sexual violence. But maybe this violence is ignored by international policies and public health interventions because the latter chose to neglect the emotional well-being of traumatized refugee communities. The *Manifesto* speaks to the "restoration of human dignity." But how can this goal be achieved when refugees live in the dark, and a significant minority of

UN and humanitarian aid officials participate in sex orgies and "sex for food"? Gender-based violence occurs because perpetrators feel and know they can get away with it. What is new, however, is that the UN, non-governmental organizations and refugees themselves have shined a bright light on this terrible reality. We have the laws to make a real difference, when the world is ready to act.

Over the past 30 years as director of one of America's first refugee clinics serving our nation's poorest citizens, I have witnessed a chronic discomfort in society with the poor, mentally ill patient. The care to poor psychiatrically ill patients has improved dramatically with an enormous expansion in inpatient and outpatient services; private and public dollars spent on mental health care; and the number and types of psychiatric practitioners. The quest for mental health parity with mental diagnoses from insurance providers is a further advancement. Yet, in spite of the enormous exploration in the scientific study of mental disorders, as well as the greater availability of effective psychiatric programs over the past half century, mental health services for the poor remain in disarray. The chronic mentally ill die ten years earlier than they did a decade ago; and public stigma towards them has been on the rise. The contradictions of psychiatry as a scientific practice are many as experienced firsthand by our refugee clinic. The repressive social forces which impair psychiatric patients' efforts to normalize their lives today include:

1 The dominant role of biological explanation for mental illness orients psychiatric treatment; the emphasis on diagnosis without treatment goals; the use of drugs without supporting therapies.
2 Professional expectations that certain patients are resistant to treatment or incapable of benefiting from professional care and/or psychological therapies.
3 The devaluation of the human capacity of patients to recover in spite of serious disabling symptoms and associated medical illnesses.

4 Neglect of the social embeddedness of the patient and an appreciation that emotional distress is a terminal end point of lack of adequate food, shelter, housing, schooling and unsafe living environment.
5 Bewilderment as to the central therapeutic role of the trauma story in the life of mainstream American patients who have suffered domestic violence, racial and economic oppression, and other social tragedies and the refugee newcomer who has suffered mass violence and torture.

These professional and social prejudices, well known in the mental health field, underscore the bias that those individuals we deem "economically redundant," whether due to social class, race, ethnicity, or gender, are "unworthy" of society's medical and social support. In reality, those who actually need the "most" get the "least" fulfilling Julian Hart's *inverse care law of medicine.*

Three decades of caring for poor newly arrived refugees to the United States, many of whom had been tortured, has been a continuously long-term battle to turn the *inverse care law* upside down by giving the "most" to the "least." It has been a great battle supported by local communities, inspired clinicians and policy makers, and patients to thrive in an administrative and financial environment that has continuously strived to push the clinics to the margins of mainstream care through policies and funding that, if not resisted, would have resulted in a "slow death by asphyxiation." As the American sociologist Kingsley Davis stated in 1938 in his famous essay, "Mental Hygiene and the Class Structure":

> [The] mental hygienist [i.e., modern-day psychiatrists] will ignore the dilemma. He will continue to be unconscious of his basic preconceptions at the same time that he keeps on professing objective knowledge. He will disregard his lack of preventive success as an accident, a lag, and not as an intrinsic destiny. All because his social function is not that of a scientist but that of a practicing moralist in a scientific, mobile world.

These moments of revelation led to a revolutionary and surprising conclusion: empathic failure is the bedrock of human aggression and violence. Extraordinary new advances in the neurosciences support this assertion. Empathy is a biological miracle that is "hard-wired" into all of us. It is easy to speculate why from an evolutionary point of view. Human beings are inherently capable of understanding and appreciating – getting into the mind and soul – of all other human beings and, in fact, all living creatures. Maybe even the inanimate earth itself. Italian scientists have demonstrated the biological basis of empathy in primates. Thousands of mirror neurons exist in the brain that are already pre-coded to respond "empathically" to people and events in the natural world. For example, when we witness someone burning his hand, mirror neurons fire so that we simultaneously feel this pain in ourselves. As William James, the great American psychologist and philosopher stated 100 years ago, the pain of others is our pain. Intuitively, we all know that the emotional experiences of our friends and our children resonate in us; the illnesses of the patient resonate in the doctor; the trauma stories of the torture survivors penetrate deeply into our emotional core. Are there mirror neurons for all basic human experiences? While we do not know for sure, the probability is, yes, there are. Carl Jung speculated on this a half century ago when he described a collective unconsciousness that unites all the living and deceased members of the human community into a collective shared experience, passed on from generation to generation. Jung's concept was rejected as Lamarckian, that is, a model of social evolution which asserts that social experiences are passed to the newborn infant at birth. But now we know that the collective unconscious is in the mirror neurons. This network of empathic integration allows us to move beyond the individualism of Martin Buber's extension of *I–It*, the common subject–object relationship to the *I–Thou*, the subject to subject interaction to an *I–Everybody*, a subject to community connectedness. The ancient Greek philosopher Heraclitus endorsed this reality over 2000 years ago when he stated that a man in sleep is self-enclosed and abandoned to himself, but he awakens to a life with other human beings, within a world common to all:

All things are one.

By which he meant:

[U]nless people reflect on their experience and examine themselves, they are condemned to live a dreamlike existence and to remain out of touch with the formula that governs and explains the nature of things. (A.A. Long, in *The Shorter Routledge Encyclopedia of Philosophy*, edited by Edward Craig, 2005)

This love of the spider's web of life within the *I–Thou* and *I–Everybody* world of human relationships is well known to cancer patients and others confronted with death who have been thrown into the timelessness of an all-encompassing world. This empathic love affair with life I have termed *empathophilia*. A new name sometimes has to be coined to emphasize a new perspective and a new way of seeing and behaving.

The stories of the UN official, the Human Rights Director, and the refugee clinic show another universal truth: empathy is easily overridden by human and social drives, especially greed, fear, and envy. Sigmund Freud attempted to explain human aggression by positing a Death Drive (*Thanatos*) towards death and destruction. In Freud's theory, the conflict between *Eros*, the Life Force, and *Thanatos*, the Death Force, leads to human aggression as the displacement of human destructive energy on to others in order to "save" ourselves. This theory shows us how ordinary people can displace their aggression so readily on to others.

From a broader sociocultural perspective, empathy can be easily overridden by personal and political forces, such as historical–political resentments (e.g., ethnic cleansing in Bosnia of Muslim Bosnians by Serbian Bosnians), and social oppression (e.g., racism). Powerful emotions such as fear, envy and greed can fuel our destructive actions. Fear is often behind empathic failure as human beings objectify others into an "enemy" that is in need of being contained and even eliminated (e.g., use of child soldiers in Uganda by the Lord's Resistance Army to kill their own parents). Envy is a powerful toxin to empathy as we must own, control, and eventually destroy that which we feel is better than ourselves and makes us feel inferior (e.g., sexual exploitation of women). Greed is the insatiable appetite for power manifested through material and social aggrandizement.

Thanatos, the Death Drive, and related forces of envy, fear, and greed, dominate empathy through its main instrument of aggression – humiliation. The goal of violent acts, regardless of intensity, is the same, that is, to create the emotional state of humiliation. During a training event I was conducting in Peru, an experienced local psychologist asked how I would deal clinically with the following scenario. She describes her therapy with a woman in the Andes who had been a victim of political oppression by Shining Path terrorists and was currently being abused by her husband who was beating her daily as well as forcing her to have sex. Poor, and living with her husband and son and two daughters, she felt privileged to receive the support of her psychologist. Slowly, over time, her husband joined the counseling sessions and recognized the terrible impact he was having on a devoted wife and his children. The domestic violence came to a halt and the couple left for a brief holiday with their daughters, leaving the older son behind to take care of their farm. Upon return, the mother walked into the kitchen and looked out the window. Her adolescent son was hanging dead from a tree in the garden. Her brother had killed his nephew over a minor land dispute. The mother, overwhelmed with grief, returned to therapy with her psychologist. Shortly thereafter, the mayor of the village sent a policeman to tell the psychologist that if she assisted her client in pressing charges against her brother (a friend of the mayor), she would be hurt. The case was never prosecuted.

During acts of violence there is a complete absence of love, affection, and empathy. As in the last circle of Dante's *Inferno*, the world is completely frozen in ice due to the total absence of love brought about through the actions of the three great betrayers of

history – Judas, Brutus, and Cassius – who are being chewed eternally in Satan's mouth. This Peruvian story was so disturbing that it initially could not be discussed professionally as a clinical case but had to be responded to in a human way. The incomprehensible pain of the mother and the simultaneous despair of the psychologist had to be first acknowledged. In this story, the nature of violent feelings of humiliation is fully revealed. The brother strikes down his sister and her family though a human action that is beyond belief. The state of humiliation created in the victim by the perpetrator is characterized by feelings of physical and mental weakness and inferiority, uncleanliness and shame, of spiritual worthlessness and guilt, and of moral repulsiveness to others, including a god or higher being. A cruel brother caused more hurt for his sister and her family than could have ever been created by the Shining Path.

Recognizing humiliation as the major tool of violent perpetrators can lend coherence to many situations that are overwhelmed by strong emotions of anger and despair. Sharing this insight with survivors from all walks of life who have experienced trafficking, sexual abuse, domestic violence, and state-sanctioned violence has led to a clarity of causes and effects. This was demonstrated in a noteworthy meeting with survivors of the Innocence Project, ex-prisoners who had been falsely incarcerated for an average of fifteen years for crimes they had not committed. These groups of survivors, mostly African-American men, had been released due to new DNA evidence. The usual scenario was an arrest of a teenager and long-term incarceration finally ending after the new DNA testing proved them innocent. Almost universally, all were thrown out of prison with little recognition by government officials that a human being's life had been wasted in jail due to inadequate evidence. Some were only given a few dollars, and a new set of clothes, and told to leave and go home. Illogically, they were now considered criminals because they had spent so much time in jail, i.e., in spite of their innocence, they had been transformed into criminals. The feelings of humiliation of these jail survivors were extreme with each one having a powerful anecdote to tell. One stated, for example, she had never recovered from being filmed on television where her children and family saw her being led away in shackles during a wrongful arrest. Surprisingly, after recognizing the centrality of humiliation, the conversation turned to acts of forgiveness and redemption that has allowed them to cope with their situation.

These revelations helped me witness something at the deepest level essential to healing a violent world. Freud hinted at this in his belief that the existence of "hatred" is older than "love" and that the death drive was due to the desire to return to a pre-organic inanimate state. Maybe Freud was not so far off. Philosophers since Plato through Kant and Sartre have recognized an ideal place or *noumena* behind reality that cannot be comprehended by the senses or empirically proven to exist, from which human beings derive their life-giving energy. The birth of human consciousness has led to the fall from a pure state of being which Kant and Sartre called "being-in-itself." I believe human beings are alienated from nature and can only return to this ideal state, not through violence and destruction as postulated by Freud, but through the creation of beauty. Indigenous people like the Navajos acknowledge this as central to the healing experience, as revealed in this healing chant.

> Today I will walk out, today everything evil will leave me,
> I will be as I was before, I will have a cool breeze over my body.
> I will have a light body, I will be happy forever, nothing will hinder me.
>
> I walk with beauty before me. I walk with beauty behind me.
> I walk with beauty below me. I walk with beauty above me.
> I walk with beauty all around me. My words will be beautiful.
>
> In beauty all day long may I walk.
> Through the returning seasons, may I walk.

> With beauty before me may I walk.
> With beauty behind me may I walk.
> With beauty below me may I walk.
> With beauty above me may I walk.
> With beauty all around me may I walk.
>
> In old age, wandering on a trail of beauty,
> Lively, may I walk.
> In old age wandering on a trail of beauty,
> Living again, may I walk.
> My words will be beautiful.

Someday the neurosciences will reveal that the antidote to human aggression is beauty and that no healing can occur without beauty. A model of beautiful healing environments, going back to the great Greek temples of the god of medicine, Aescalapius, are ready at hand. Even now, our sterile and inhumane intensive care units and hospital wards are slowly being transformed into beautiful therapeutic spaces.

I have fought against treating poor patients such as refugee and torture survivors in clinical settings that are filthy and degrading to patients and staff. For over 30 years, a battle our clinic has won has been to treat patients in a space filled with art from their own indigenous cultures. This battle still goes on today, not only in the impoverished refugee camps but in rich hospital settings. Let the patient beware of the quality of care if the medical clinic has stained rugs, unpainted walls, broken chairs, and an unhygienic toilet. It only takes $200 to buy art posters, plants, a broom, and a wash cloth, and fill a clean clinic with beautiful art made by patients and their communities. Similarly, I have witnessed in the most destitute refugee camps, local residents transform barren spaces into magnificent places of healing. In contrast, it baffles me to be in psychiatrists' offices, they sit in completely empty rooms except for a desk and a chair, caring for emotionally distressed people.

There must be radical change in how we prevent violence as well as heal its damaging effects. The empathic transformation of daily relationships including our interaction in schools, churches, the workplace, and in our social and public policies must occur. At the turn of the nineteenth century, Italian Futurist painters glorified the cleansing and purification of human society, through war. As Filippo Tommaso Marinetti, the intellectual leader of the Futurist movement declared, "we will glorify war – the world's only hygiene – militarism, patriotism, the destructive gesture of freedom bringers, beautiful ideas worth dying for … ." Ultimately, these artists became advocates of World War I and supporters of the rise of Italian Fascism. Medical institutions today are caught up in a similar glorification of medical machines, invasive surgeries, and expensive drugs. There is a glorification of the "isolated mind" and the "isolated body part." The patient is a "kidney," cancer is a "product line," and patients are "consumers." Beauty and empathy are marginalized as alternative forms of healing. Expensive and often needless surgeries (e.g., triple cardiac bypass surgery) are elevated over comparably effective human-based clinical practices such as diet, exercise, and stress reduction. Those who treat the poor, the homeless, and the refugee are marginalized in medical ghettos as foolish but dedicated people who are doing "God's work." Social factors that contribute to medical and psychiatric illnesses are excluded from medical care because of a false belief that there is nothing medicine can do about poverty, racism, and violence. This foolish statement is, of course, an ideological belief based on the worship of technology and wealth.

A great revolution in human relationships is occurring in our modern age around the World Wide Web. Internet and cellphone technology has created an amazing opportunity for easy access to unlimited knowledge and instantaneous communication with each other. It has also increased the danger of human exploitation and oppression. Similar to the great historic anxiety brought on by past innovations, our rapidly accelerating "wired world" is creating great social challenges. While the internet can generate great human solidarity (as evidenced by the massive demonstrations orchestrated by the high school students of Marjory Stoneman Douglas High School to eliminate gun violence), it has also created an upsurge in bullying on social media, the spreading of violence as a form of entertainment, and the disengagement of users from nature and from each other. Emotional intelligence may be on the decline and lack of empathic skills on the rise. As MIT Professor Sherry Turkle, a life-long researcher on technology and social relationships stated:

Technology is seductive when what it offers meets our human vulnerability. And as it turns out, we are very vulnerable indeed. We are lonely but fearful of intimacy. Digital connections and the sociable robot may offer the illusion of companionship without the demands of friendship. Our networked life allows us to hide from each other, even as we are tethered to each other. We'd rather text than talk.

While we are witnessing an ascendance in levels of social connections, we are also witnessing a decline in deep listening, respect for others, and a deterioration of meaningful personal relationships with families, friends, and our local communities. There is real danger of disconnecting and disengaging from the human and natural world. The computer (or robot) cannot answer the basic questions of our existence: "Who am I? What is my journey? And how do I give meaning to my life?"

By embracing our biologically based precondition for empathy and by operationalizing personal actions and policies based on *empathophilia*, and the creation of beauty in our healing environments, we can stop the deleterious effects of human violence and create truly therapeutic healing environments. From the great whales and redwoods to the tiniest insect and bacterial cell, we are all linked together by one shared ancestral past. As the great Native American statesman of the Nez Perce, Chief Joseph, stated over 100 years ago: "The earth is the mother of all people, and all people should have equal rights upon it."

This *Manifesto* is a call to action for each and every person to enter fully into a relationship with the miracle of our shared existence with plants, animals, humans, and the earth itself.

AFTERWORD

Marjorie Agosín

THROUGHOUT HISTORY, THE POET has been able to illustrate the indescribable and has been able to illuminate the malignancy of our time, weaving metaphors and images with the enchantment of lyricism. Poetry belongs to the realm of beauty and transformation, also to the sacredness of the human voice. We have all began as poets, describing our world and our common humanity, singing to its beauty and to its sorrows.

This historical *Manifesto* explores how communities can heal the catastrophe of our times through the pursuit of beauty and truth. Poetry has the task of repairing and mending our own individual and collective histories, and the power to heal our own suffering.

These poems were written as a response to Richard Mollica's *Manifesto*, creating a magical alchemy between the voice of a physician and a poet trying to reimagine our world and use poetical thinking as well as healing to its highest power. The poems are intended to transform the bleak realities of our time into a world filled with grace, beauty, and poetry. These poems can be viewed as golden threads of hope. As scraps of memory and mostly as a reciprocity between physician, poet, and reader. I invite all of you to enter the thresholds of art through the reading of this *Manifesto vis-à-vis* the poetry that was inspired by it in a world filled with violence. I invite the reader to join us in the celebration of creativity and in the reciprocity between readers and writers.

I myself grew up in a country that venerates, and murders, its poets. I came of age in the midst of a military dictatorship in Chile that dismantled our democratic ways and destroyed our civil society. Nevertheless, the people continued to write, and to paint the walls of the city with verses of hope and resistance. People lived inside themselves and in the beautiful republic of the imagination – I understood that as a poet. I could inspire others to join the world of lyrical language and create a reality of beauty and possibility, not the realm of violence and hatred.

Art is the true revolution of the human spirit; it endures, and it inspires to live in dignity. I inspire you to read the *Manifesto* and these sparkling poems with an open soul. Read them at loud or to yourself. Read them with the faith that we will find one another in beauty and in art and that the impossible becomes possible when we engage in the voice of poetry which is the voice of our world.

PEARLS OF OBSERVATIONS ON OUR VIOLENT WORLD

Marjorie Agosín

Night

Night cascaded over the darkness of time
Devouring the break of dawn
The light no longer seemed to be of this
    world
And death bestowed mercy upon the bodies
Without names, without a past.

Haven

Only the earth gave shelter to the bones
    of the defenseless
Only the earth provided a haven and peace
To the humiliated.

Fearless

If you could just heed the song of others
The passing voices of those
Who search for a blue door
A piece of warm bread on a generous table.

If you could just be fearless
And open a door without
Shadows and doubts
Only a blue door
Only once.

New light

The deceitful, moving water
At the edge of night
Water safer than the cities filled with
Bodies numbed by certain death.
Believe me when I tell you that although
    sinister
The water offered the illusion of an
    arrival
At a New Harbor where kind-hearted beings
    awaited.
My voice opened like a nocturnal
    butterfly
Transforming into a chorus of voices
And the darkness impacted by these new
    sounds
Gave way to a new light.

Stillness

Never again to rescue bodies among the
    debris
And the complicity of perverse stillness.

Life

Only a flicker of vulnerable life, an
    unimaginable
Glorious rhapsody

Our boy

The body of the marooned child lying on
   the sand
Is covered with seaweed by the village
   women
Who also close his sky-blue eyes.
What they saw is true
A dead child washed up on the shore
With his party clothes and patent
   leather shoes.

The travelers

Before us, the grief
The lifeless body
Of a child
With unfulfilled hopes
And dreams.
There was no one to rescue them
Those who remained silent, had moved
To more prosperous cities
They didn't reach the shore
No one received them
Only deceptive and merciful death
Godforsaken travelers.

Hope

You will begin to confide in strangers
The ones who welcomed you and
Offered you hope and water.

Mother

Gasping, howling,
The woman with the amputated hand appears
Unable to comb her daughter's hair.
Her body, a world in cinders.
A woman sobs
And arrives with a bleeding heart
And her hair in flames.

Thirst

You yearn for a glass of water
The light of a day with a clear destiny
Time without haste
Your hand caresses mine
Your language is also mine
We are a single voice
Amid the rainfall.

The dinghy

The dark waters
The stormy sea
An insecure raft
By the black water and
Ravenous sea.
New life on the coast
Death in the dark water
Hope to reach the shore
To abandon the raging sea and
Life amid the flames.

The departed

We have slowly gathered the garments of
   the departed
Amid the drifting sand and cracked earth
Where the figures and
Bones of the dead lay.
We have slowly gathered the garments of
   the departed
Lives among the ashes
Stories muzzled in the great silence of
   history.

The light

Once again you will feel the delightful
   presence of beloved objects
The sun filtering through your hands
Your bare feet touching the earth
   undisturbed by bombs.
And soon you will recognize the songs of
   nocturnal birds
Showing the way to your new home
Where everyone waits for you
And the mirrors fill with light.

Escape

Someday no one will flee from home
We shall walk secure in our cities and
Be acquainted with blossoming gardens.
There will be no shadows or oblivion
We will be like the rivers
Without borders
Without walls.

You shall walk amid the fresh blades of
   grass and
Your bare feet will recognize the kindness
   of the dew
You shall not fear a new war or
The face of death.

(Translated by Celeste Kostopulos-Cooperman.)

ON BEAUTY AND THE OBLIGATION TO CARE

COMMENTARY

Nisha Sajnani

AS I REFLECTED ON these manifestos and poems, I had to ask myself "What does beauty have to do with the obligation to care? Is it a frivolous pursuit for those with the means to distract themselves from daily travails or is it necessary to our survival?" As someone concerned, both personally and professionally, with the safety, dignity, and health of individuals and communities, I am invested in what beauty is and does in a time where the realities of cruelty, violence, and exclusion are dismissed as relative "truthiness" or, worse still, justified as being hard-wired in human beings. What claim can beauty make in a morally ambiguous world? I take, as my starting point, a line from Richard Mollica's first manifesto in which he declares that "except in beauty there is no healing". Beauty is what permeates through spaces and relationships where we find hope and healing. But how do Dr. Mollica, a physician, and Professor Agosín, a poet, work together to make this claim?

A Call to Attention

Let us begin with a common definition of beauty as qualities in a person or thing that gives pleasure to the senses. Beauty arrests us. It lifts us out of the quotidian, invites contemplation, and may be necessary to our survival. For example, the presence of arrowheads constructed of rare, impractical materials in early civilization were argued as evidence of the role of beauty in stimulating the propagation of the species. The idea here being that access to such singularities signaled wealth and good health to a potential

mate. At first glance, this argument seems to undo any obligation that beauty may have to ethics for, in this Darwinian equation, the purpose of beauty is to ensure survival not equity. However, from this evolutionary perspective, we can also deduce an argument for diversity as organisms continually adapt to their environments, and the variety of environments that exists promotes a diversity of organisms adapted to them. It is precisely the uniqueness – the difference – of an encounter with someone or something that compels attention, adaptation, and transformation. When we experience a poem, photograph, film, play, or story that reflects our struggles, we are given the opportunity to better see ourselves and each other. We are given a chance to adapt in response to the particular and the universal.

A manifesto is an urgent call to attention and a refusal to accept the *status quo*. Mollica opens his first manifesto with three words: SEEING REALITY CLEARLY. These words are a demand, an invitation, and a nod to the artist Piero della Francesca whose discovery of perspective in painting revolutionized the art form. Mollica urges the reader to gain perspective and hold on to our ideals with him through his use of the word *we*: We who know that the pain of the world is too much to bear yet "do not give up our dream for a more loving and peaceful humanity." He articulates twelve carefully chosen points that pronounce a new code of ethics centered on a brave acknowledgment of truths that we must not only understand but also be affected by in order to move from knowledge to action.

Aesthetic Ambiguity and Aesthetic Distance

Agosín's poem, *A Woman Dreams Between the Thresholds* follows Mollica's first manifesto. This placement is important because, like Mollica, she implicates her readers. She writes:

> You could have been her
> The girl amid the rubble
> The girl dissolved by the haze of fire and hatred
> But, you were not her.
> You turned the corner of good fortune
>
> Luck and its premonitions accompanied you.
> But, could you have been her?
> The girl amid the rubble?

Here, Agosín brings us into imaginative contact with the suffering of a young girl "dissolved" by degradation. I read this stanza as a personal call to account for my accidental safety. Her questions tap away at our mental defenses against the possibility of such horror affecting our own families and homes. Mollica writes: "Only through imagination can healing occur. Healing is the imagination to heal." Agosín responds with images that transport us into an imaginary world where we are able to experience our own fear, grief, and longing.

What makes her poetry effective is, in part, related to the ambiguity that clings to the images that she creates. Her images reflect and prompt *aesthetic ambiguity* which facilitates multiple meanings in the imagination of the reader in each unique encounter. Paradoxically, it is the space between the lines, the incompleteness, and approximation that stimulates a search for meaning and coherence. Her metaphors create *aesthetic distance* allowing the reader to engage with both thought and feeling. She works together with Mollica to move us from the head to the heart and back again.

Beauty in the Empathic Double Helix of the Therapeutic Encounter

In Mollica's second manifesto, he writes of the vitality that arises from "listening and understanding with deep appreciation." He writes of the beauty of conversation, a word that comes from the Latin *conversare*, which means to "dwell with" and "turn together." He illuminates the centrality of the healer and the patient turning together in an empathic double helix. The DNA of the healing relationship is found in the smallest units of our social interaction: our gestures, glances, sounds, and our words. He refers to woundedness of not only the patient but the healer as well who both learn from each other and who both need and empathic space to share the stories that they carry.

In the hands of the those seeking and offering healing, crafting stories from our lives can help us to make connections out of chaos, to weave seemingly disparate events and experiences into a coherent form. This allows us to make meaning and it allows us to communicate something of our inner experience to another human being. Stories transport us. They allow us to raise questions, present unresolved conflicts, weigh the consequences of potential activity, resolve crises, claim strengths, inhabit new possibilities and, as Mollica writes, move us closer to an empathic horizon with another. Our narratives can help us to better understand and be understood by others which can help us create and sustain social support. Such networks of care have been well documented to be a highly significant predictor of good physical and psychological health and a potent protective factor when faced with stress. The duty of the listener is to feel, think, and respond. Thus, the listener is accountable to the teller. Herein lies the problem and the solution. Why risk listening when it means that we will need to let ourselves be affected, be called into presence, and may have to change something in response? To deny the consequences of a telling still constitutes a response. To this, Mollica urges us to be unafraid, for the stories that we hear and tell have profound consequences for how we relate to our environment and to each other. They make all the difference in whether we see another living being as one to be dominated quickly or as an equal worthy of time, dignity, and respect.

Agosín's second poem is a tribute to healers who are able to practice the art of listening to the "sealed up words, the motions of silence." In four stanzas, she describes the therapeutic encounter and calls us to listen to the whole body. She rescues the healer from the ruins of humiliation and enrolls them as a generous "festival" where they bring light.

Linking Personal Healing and Social Justice

Mollica's third manifesto returns to the concept of justice and social healing which he claims "cannot occur without concern for personal healing." This healing must not be limited to physical health but must facilitate self-determination. He calls upon Platonic notions of ideal Beauty, distinct because of its harmony and balance, as the conduit to fairness and equity. Drawing on lessons learned working with women in Gujarat, he quotes:

> Health is a personal and social state of balance and well-being in which people feel strong, active, wise, and worthwhile; where their diverse capacities and rhythms are valued, where they may decide and choose, express themselves, and move about freely.

He reminds us that the path to this ideal balance is, once again, through storytelling and story-listening because to share our stories is to share our truths which should be "collected and archived for all to read without censorship." He ends this third manifesto with a shift towards love for each other and for our natural environment.

Agosín's third poem calls justice into cities in ruin to restore the presence of beauty with the sinew of words like *solidarity*, *empathy*, and *goodness*. She, too, recognizes the need to heal the lovers, the children, the streets, and the cities affected by war. Social healing is again linked to personal healing evidenced by our actions with one another. Beauty is expressed in our capacity to welcome, confide, and care for one another.

Towards the Ideal City

To conclude, the doctor and the poet have written a dream with instructions on how to enter and inhabit the Ideal City. They seek to salvage us from the decay of compassion and care by asking us to imagine the possibility of beauty in the spaces and relationships that we participate in. They ask us to move without fear into each other's embrace so that we might experience the fullest expression of human creativity and dignity.

How do we translate these ideas about beauty and justice into the material messiness of our everyday lives where so much care is needed? Like Agosín's blue door in her final poem, we must begin by being brave enough to walk through believing that another world is possible. The spaces that we create to share our truths, to become ourselves with each other, are carved out by our own listening. This call to empathic presence with each other is the foundation for healing. Such spaces, where people are invited to tell their stories, sing their songs, dance their dances, read their poems, and perform their lives, invite bravery, playfulness, dialogue, and love. Here, aesthetics become relational in that our expressions reflect and prompt a sense of our interconnectedness or what Martin Luther King Jr. referred to as our Beloved Community.

Further Reading

Bullough, E. (1912). "Psychic Distance" as a factor in art and as an aesthetic principle. *British Journal of Psychology* 5: 87–117.

Dutton, D. (2009). *The Art Instinct: Beauty, pleasure, & human evolution*. Oxford: Oxford University Press.

Green, M.C. and Brock, T. (2000). The role of transportation in the persuasiveness of public narratives. *Journal of Personality and Social Psychology* 79(5): 701–21.

Kaplan, A. and Kris, E. (1947). Esthetic ambiguity. *Philosophy and Phenomenological Research* 8(3): 415–35.

King, M.L. (1963). *Why We Can't Wait*. London: Penguin Books.

Landy, R. (1997). Drama therapy and distancing: Reflections on theory and clinical application. *Arts in Psychotherapy* 23(5): 367–3.

Ozbay, F., Johnson, D.C., Dimoulas, E., Morgan, C.A., Charney, D. and Southwick, S. (2007). Social support and resilience to stress: From neurobiology to clinical practice. *Psychiatry (Edgmont)* 4(5): 35–40.

RELATIONSHIPS: THE LIGHTHOUSES OF OUR GENERATION

REFLECTIONS ON THE MANIFESTOS

Hanna Solomon and Chris Mollica

"Quando un'alba o un tramonto non ci danno più emozioni, significa che l'anima è malata."
"When a sunrise or a sunset do not evoke feelings in us anymore, it means that the soul is sick."

Roberto Gervaso

AN URGENT MATTER HAS brought healers of all kinds together. The visionaries in this *Manifesto* urge us to stop and face this crisis of alienation from one another that humankind is experiencing. They implore us to stop and dwell in the moment. To reflect and move towards change. To hold ourselves accountable for the positive influence that every individual can make. We must reach in for our innate, in Dr. Figley's words, "sense of healing" and empathy. However, kidnapped by the current of this fast paced, self-centered, individualistic, and demanding lifestyle, societies have forgotten how to float with the admiration, kindness, and curiosity that they once carried in their innocence. We have stopped "invoking" the empathy that dwells within all of us. While growing, our innocence is chipped away and molded into grotesque statues carved by an unjust and violent world.

As Dr. Mollica passionately states, human empathy can only be recalled by love. And in a world clouded by violence and hatred, we must force ourselves to push away from our comfort and seek that which inspires respect and love for one another. The one thing that can dull the pain of these extreme situations is Nature's beauty.

In the presence of a sunset, people from all walks of life stop and admire the surreal spectrum of colors floating before them. In the words of Edmund Burke, this awe-inspiring beauty is the ultimate sublime that suspends all else. For that moment in which we find ourselves in the presence of such grandeur, we are placed in a state of utter tranquility. The wilderness' beauty transcends time and *status quo*. It is not the state of horror that Burke refers to, on the contrary, it is the state of awakening. A window in which our hearts and minds are open to new things, emotions, ideas, and dreams. This moment blurs all previous burdens and prejudice. It suspends time, allowing a glimpse of a different and optimistic future, uncharted by hatred or sorrow from the past. It is this short moment of utter freedom that we must capture and learn to lengthen. It is only by mastering this tranquility that we can allow ourselves to relearn how to love, to be kind, and to be empathetic to one another. It is not an easy task to remove the stubborn certainties that have built a brick wall around our hearts. Nevertheless, we have witnessed time and time again, that healers have the ability to dismantle that wall. They have acquired the strength to put away their fears and prejudice so that their endeavors can bring about the future they envisioned in their state of tranquility.

This *Manifesto* is the lighthouse which reminds us to strive for our visions and never stop dreaming.

Hanna Solomon

THERE IS A DREAM as blue and pure as the ocean that we all strive for. A dream of family and friends, a gratifying role in society, vibrant green grass, an abundance of fruit, and innocent, genuine trees towering over head protecting us from the rain while still allowing us to feel the calming and cleansing sensation of every drop.

This dream combines our care for our loved ones and our search for personal meaning. It is not a means to an end and it takes on a different form for all of us.

In the world today we are so stressed with challenges for survival, meeting deadlines, and for choosing right over wrong. We are pressured into being the best that we can be at all costs. As a consequence, we are shoved into living in isolation defined by a desperate search for the next best thing. We are shoved and pushed towards the end.

Nonetheless, within all of us is a dream of the ocean's waves and of the whales that sing harmoniously to each other in increasingly complex languages and dance together while they swim. And like the whales, deep down we know that we all have a life to live, not an end to reach. When we are focused on reaching the end, which is set in black and white, we consequently lose the color of the dream. We lose freedom, and in some ways life itself.

Within this *Manifesto* we argue for moving away from a black and white dream. In doing so, we acknowledge that for our dream we accept the responsibility of taking on a problem we cannot solve.

We must become the heroes and heroines of our personal and shared journeys; always fighting for something better and for more color. Along the way we create and build relationships, our anchors in life.

We cherish those relationships as lighthouses in a dark storm-ridden sea; our conversations the light on what blinds us. And in doing so, we remember that our ancestors, family, friends, neighbors, colleagues, and even our pets, support us just as we support them; our times together the ships on which we sail.

The importance of safeguarding and treasuring our relationships lies in the acknowledgment that in order to grow both sides of any relationship must change. With our dreams connecting us, our responsibility as heroes and heroines, is to continue to imagine and create a better world, to grow closer and to care for one another.

As we trust ourselves, our loved ones, our journeys, and our dreams, we discover beauty in knowing there is more to life than ourselves, more to life than one simple end.

Within our generation everyone accepts their responsibility, we all protect our dignity, we love our loved ones, and color-in our individual lives. And as Bob Marley advised each of us, knowing that we always find a way, "LIVELY UP YOURSELF."

Chris Mollica

AUTHOR BIOGRAPHIES

CHARLES FIGLEY   Dr. Figley is the Tulane University Paul Henry Kurzweg, MD Distinguished Chair in Disaster Mental Health and Associate Dean for Research, Co-Founder of Disaster Resilience Leadership Academy in the School of Social Work, and Director of the award-winning Traumatology Institute. He is a former professor at both Purdue University (1974–89) and then at Florida State University (1989–2008) and former Fulbright Fellow and Visiting Distinguished Professor at Kuwait University (2003–4).

Professor Figley received both graduate degrees from the Pennsylvania State University and his undergraduate degree from the University of Hawaii, all in the interdisciplinary field of human development. He was recently awarded by John Jay College of Criminal Justice (City University of New York) Honorary Degree in 2014.

He is founding editor of the *Journal of Traumatic Stress*, the *Journal of Family Psychotherapy*, and the American Psychological Association's journal, *Traumatology*. He is also founding editor of the book series *Death and Trauma* (Taylor & Francis), *Innovations in Psychology* (CRC Press), and continues to as editor of the *Psychosocial Stress* book series (Routledge). Professor Figley has written more than 200 scholarly works including 25 books. Most have focused on stress, particularly traumatic stress, and most recently a focus on human and systemic traumatic stress resilience. His most recent books is *First Do No Self Harm: Understanding and Promoting Physician Stress Resilience* (Oxford University Press, co-edited with P. Huggard and C. Rees, 2013). Dr. Figley is editor of the award-winning *Encyclopedia of Trauma: An Interdisciplinary Guide* (Sage References, 2012).

Among the books especially relevant to this book is *Compassion Fatigue: Coping with Secondary Traumatic Stress Disorder in Those Who Treat the Traumatized* (Brunner-Routledge, 1995) and *Treating Compassion Fatigue* (Routledge, 2002). In addition to books, Dr. Figley has published more than 160 peer-reviewed journal articles, more than 60 chapters, and more than 400 scholarly presentations and guest lectures all over the world since 1975.

His current research focuses on understanding compassion fatigue resilience and strategies for building resilience through self-care, social support, and other protective factors. At the same time, he is engaged in numerous humanitarian activities including volunteer work to stop torture, increase reproductive freedom, and stop suicides among war veterans.

NISHA SAJNANI   Nisha Sajnani is an Associate Professor of Drama Therapy, Director of the Drama Therapy Program, and on the faculty of the Educational Theatre EdD/PhD and Rehabilitation Sciences PhD program at New York University. She is also on faculty with the Harvard Program in Refugee Trauma where she lectures on the role of beauty and the arts in global mental health. Dr. Sajnani is a Canadian-born multimedia artist who works with oral histories, digital photography, video, improvisation, and performance to explore memory, identity, ethics, and place. She directed *Under Pressure* (2014), a performance collage featuring community responses to the Boston Marathon bombing, and *Lives That Matter* (2015), an ethnodrama examining racism, identity politics, and hashtag activism. Her writing has been featured in *Diverse Issues in Higher Education*, *Alt. Theatre: Cultural Diversity and the Stage*, *The Arts in Psychotheraphy*, *Applied Arts and Health*, *Canadian Theatre Review*, and the *Canadian Women's Studies* journal. Dr. Sajnani is the editor of *Drama Therapy Review*, an international, peer-reviewed journal on theatre and health. She has received several awards including the Corann Okorodudu Global Women's Advocacy Award from the American Psychological Association.

MARJORIE AGOSÍN   Marjorie Agosín is the Luella Lamer Slaner Professor of Latin American Studies at Wellesley college. She is a poet, and human rights activist, she has been recognized with numerous awards for her writing and activism and is the author of more than thirty books. Among her most recent work *I Lived on Butterfly Hill* (Atheneum Books) a young adult novel that received the Pura Belpré Award in 2015 and the poetry collections, *The White Islands* (Swan Isle Press), as well as the collection of essays, *Home*, on place and displacement (Solis Press). The government of Chile awarded her with the Gabriela Mistral Medal of honor for life achievement and she also received the Fritz Redlich Award from the Harvard Program in Refugee Trauma (HPRT). She lives in between places: in the second world of poetry and in Wellesley as well as Con Con, Chile.

CELESTE KOSTOPULOS-COOPERMAN holds an MA (1976) and a PhD (1980) in Hispanic Studies from Brown University. She is a professor in the Department of World Languages and Cultural Studies at Suffolk University, Boston, Massachusetts where she teaches all levels of Spanish language and courses in Latin American culture (including Latin American Cinema, the Latin American Short Narrative, and Translation as Art and Craft). Her translations of Latin American women's poetry have appeared in many magazines and journals.

She has also translated a number of books by Marjorie Agosín and was the recipient of the Outstanding Translation Award from the American Literary Translations Association for *Circles of Madness/ Círculos de locura: Las madres de la Plaza de Mayo* (White Pine Press, 1992). Her primary research interests are in Latin American Political and Human Rights Narratives, Gender Studies, Latin American Film, Latino Literature, and Translation Theory and Practice.

RICHARD F. MOLLICA   Richard Mollica, MD, MAR is a Professor of Psychiatry at Harvard Medical School and Director of the Harvard Program in Refugee Trauma (HPRT) at Massachusetts General Hospital. Since 1981, Dr. Mollica and HPRT have pioneered the medical and mental health care of survivors of mass violence and torture in the USA and abroad. Under Dr. Mollica's direction, HPRT conducts clinical, training, policy, and research activities for populations affected by mass violence around the world. Dr. Mollica is currently active in clinical work, research, and the development of a Global Health curriculum, focusing on trauma and recovery. The *Global Mental Health: Trauma and Recovery* certificate program is the first of its kind in global mental health and post-conflict/disaster. Dr. Mollica has published over 160 scientific manuscripts and has recently published his first book, *Healing Invisible Wounds: Paths to Hope and Recovery in a Violent World.*

CHRISTOPHER J. MOLLICA   Chris Mollica is studying to receive his doctorate in psychology from William James College in Newton, Massachusetts. He recently worked as a research assistant at the HPRT. During his time there he assisted in the coordination of HPRT's annual Global Mental Health: Trauma and Recovery Certificate program. He also participated in the preparation of a health promotion project for rural women in Liberia. Chris received a bachelor's degree in biology from Northeastern University in Boston. During his undergraduate career he studied for nearly a year at the Consiglio Nazionale delle Ricerche (National Research Council) in Porano, Italy. In addition to this experience, he completed an internship at a Cambodian health care clinic that offers both primary and behavioral health care in Long Beach, California. Currently, Chris volunteers for an afterschool program in Boston that is designed to bring kids closer to the natural world. Chris also volunteers to help run a local storytelling show for the general public two nights of every month. Chris' interests lie primarily in the use of storytelling to treat mental illness and in the intersections between the time we spend in nature and our overall well-being.

HANNA SOLOMON   Hanna Solomon is a rising senior at Tufts University. She is currently assisting at the Harvard Program in Refugee Trauma in the Liberian Women's Health Promotion Project. Hanna's interests lie in introducing and promoting emotional and mental health in underprivileged communities. As a torture survivor herself, she has presented speeches at the United Nations both in Geneva (2015 and 2016) and New York (2017) against the atrocities and injustice in her home country Eritrea. After resettling in the USA in 2012, she pursued an education in clinical psychology. During her undergraduate studies, she has worked with refugee and immigrant communities. She has interned at the International Institute of New England (IINE), an organization that helps refugees resettle in the USA, and has assisted IINE in an outreach program by telling her trauma and recovery story. She is also a volunteer tutor for immigrant families at the Welcome Project.

www.ingramcontent.com/pod-product-compliance
Lightning Source LLC
Chambersburg PA
CBHW041608260326
41914CB00012B/1419

9 7 8 1 9 1 0 1 4 6 3 4 7